P^{The}ocket Doctor

1999

The Pocket Doctor

1999

Michael S. Sherman, M.D.
Edward S. Schulman, M.D.
MCP Hahnemann School of Medicine

EDUCATIONAL COMMUNICATIONS
Mount Kisco, New York

The Pocket Doctor is intended as a quick and convenient reminder of information you have learned previously. Treatment recommendations are based on published clinical practice guidelines, reliable medical literature, and interpretation by our authors who are knowledgeable in their fields. Tables and algorithms are designed as a guide for uncomplicated patients and are not meant as a substitute for sound clinical judgement and, where appropriate, individualization of therapy. Though extensive efforts were made to assure accuracy and completeness, unerring treatment recommendations cannot be guaranteed. Moreover, *The Pocket Doctor* may contain typographical errors, omissions, and in certain instances, controversial treatment preferences of the authors.

In general, drug indications and dosages listed in *The Pocket Doctor* have been recommended in the medical literature and conform to the practices of the general medical community, rather than those of any specific institution, geographic region, or practice specialty. However, this does not imply approval of the United States Food and Drug Administration (FDA) for their use in the diseases and dosages listed. Package inserts for each drug should be consulted for the uses and dosages that are FDA approved. Also, because of constant modifications of indications and dosages, particularly of new drugs, it is necessary for the health care professional to keep abreast of such revised recommendations.

ISBN: 0-967-2263-0-9

PRINTED IN THE UNITED STATES OF AMERICA

About our web site: www.PocketDoctor.com

In recognition of the rapidity of changes in medical knowledge, we have established a free internet site, **www.PocketDoctor.com.** Currently under construction, this web site will offer the individual algorithms that appear in the book version along with annotations on critical decision points and, where available, links to references and other relevant source material. As we receive new information, guideline changes, and feedback from our readers, the editors and authors will modify individual algorithms and tables "on-line." Updates will be posted frequently. Please check this site regularly for changes. Registered users will be informed by e-mail when new material is added to the site. Downloads of new algorithms may be printed and can be sized to paste in the book. We welcome your comments and suggestions, which can be posted on the site.

Contents

Contributors

Neil Aronin MD
Professor of Medicine and Cell Biology
University of Massachusetts Medical
Center

Ausim Azizi
Associate Professor of Neurology
MCP Hahnemann School of Medicine

Jack Becker MD
Assistant Professor of Medicine
Chief, Section of Allergy
St. Christopher's Hospital for Children

Thompson K. Boyd III MD
Assistant Professor of Medicine
Chairman, Utilization Review
MCP Hahnemann School of Medicine

Harris Clearfield MD
Professor of Medicine
Division of Gastroenterology
MCP Hahnemann School of Medicine

Stephen Bulova MD
Professor of Medicine
Division of Hematology/Oncology
MCP Hahnemann School of Medicine

James Conroy DO, FACP, FACOI
Professor of Medicine
Division of Hematology/Oncology
MCP Hahnemann School of Medicine

Jane Doszpoly MA, RD, CNSD
Department of Nutrition Services
Hahnemann University Hospital

Mary Elmer RN, CCRN, CRNP
Jefferson Medical College

Sol Epstein M.D.
Head, Division of Endocrinology and
Metabolism
Director of Osteoporosis and Bone
Metabolism
MCP Hahnemann School of Medicine

Babak Etemad MD
Assistant Professor of Medicine
Director, GI Diagnostic Laboratory
MCP Hahnemann School of Medicine

Pierre B. Fayad M.D.
Associate Professor of Neurology
Yale University

Amy Chernoff Fuchs
Assistant Professor of Medicine
Division of Infectious Diseases
MCP Hahnemann School of Medicine

Barry Fuchs MD
Assistant Professor of Medicine
Chief, Section of Critical Care Medicine
Director, Medical Intensive Care Units
MCP Hahnemann School of Medicine

Jeffrey Glassroth MD
Love Professor and Chair
Department of Medicine
University of Wisconsin-Madison Medical
School

Jonathan E. Gottlieb MD
Associate Professor of Medicine
Division of Pulmonary and Critical Care
Jefferson Medical College

Scott Hessen MD
Assistant Professor of Medicine
Division of Cardiology
MCP Hahnemann School of Medicine

Susan Hoch MD
Associate Professor of Medicine
Lupus and Arthritis Center
MCP Hahnemann School of Medicine

David M. Hoenig MD
Director of Endourology
MCP Hahnemann School of Medicine

Steven L. Hubert MD
Assistant Professor of Dermatology
MCP Hahnemann School of Medicine

Mercedes P. Jacobson MD
Director, Epilepsy Center
MCP Hahnemann School of Medicine

Draga Jichici HBSc, MD, FRCPC
Assistant Professor of Neurology
MCP Hahnemann School of Medicine

Margaret Khouri MD
Associate Professor of Medicine
Division of Gastroenterology
Texas Tech University Health Science
Center at Odessa

Robert Kotloff MD
Associate Professor of Medicine
Pulmonary and Critical Care Division
University of Pennsylvania School of
Medicine

Thomas Kowalski MD
Assistant Professor of Medicine
Director of Endoscopy
Division of Gastroenterology
MCP Hahnemann School of Medicine

David Kountz, MD
Associate Professor of Medicine
Associate Dean for Postgraduate
Education
UMDNJ-Robert Wood Johnson Medical
School

Steven Kutalek MD
Associate Professor of Medicine
Division of Cardiology
MCP Hahnemann School of Medicine

David Lang MD
Associate Professor of Medicine
Director, Division of Allergy and
Immunology
MCP Hahnemann School of Medicine

Alyssa A. LeBel MD
Director, Neurology Pain Service
Hahnemann Hospital
MCP Hahnemann School of Medicine

David C. Lee, MD, FAAEM
Assistant Professor
Department of Emergency Medicine
NYU School of Medicine
North Shore University Hospital

Frank Leone MD
Director, Medical Respiratory Intensive
Care Unit
Thomas Jefferson University Hospital

Carlos M. Martinez MD
Assistant Professor of Medicine
Department of Family Practice
Bella Vista Hospital, Mayagüez, Puerto Rico

A. Scott Mathis, Pharm. D.
Assistant Clinical Professor
Rutgers College of Pharmacy
Rutgers University

Joseph McClellen MD
Associate Professor of Medicine
Cardiology Division
University of Pennsylvania School of
Medicine

Arthur Meltzer MD
Clinical Assistant Professor of Medicine
Cardiology Division
MCP Hahnemann School of Medicine

Geno Merli MD, FACP
Ludwig A. Kind
Professor and Director, Division of
Internal Medicine
Vice Chairman of Primary Care
Jefferson Medical College

John Morgan MD
Associate director, Cardiovascular
Disease Prevention Center
Jefferson Medical College

Thomas J. Nasca MD, FACP
Professor of Medicine
Associate Dean
Jefferson Medical College

Michael Niederman M.D.
Professor of Medicine
SUNY Stony Brook
Chief, Pulmonary and Critical Care
Division
Winthrop University Hospital

Harold I. Palevsky MD
Chief, Pulmonary and Critical Care
Division
Presbyterian Medical Center
Associate Professor of Medicine
University of Pennsylvania School of
Medicine

Herbert Patrick MD
Clinical Associate Professor of Medicine
Medical Director, Respiratory Care
Thomas Jefferson University Hospital

Donald G. Raible MD
Associate Professor of Medicine
Division of Pulmonary and Critical Care
MCP Hahnemann School of Medicine

James Reynolds MD
Professor of Medicine and Chief,
Division of Gastroenterology and
Hepatology
MCP Hahnemann School of Medicine

Leslie Rose MD
Professor of Medicine
Division of Endocrinology and
Metabolism
MCP Hahnemann School of Medicine

Daniel Rukstalis M.D.
Associate Professor of Surgery and
Pathology
Urology Division
MCP Hahnemann School of Medicine

Jamie Ellen Siegel MD
Assistant Professor of Medicine
Hematology Division
UMDNJ-Robert Wood Johnson Medical
School

Edward S. Schulman M.D.
Professor of Medicine and
Associate Chairman for Research
MCP Hahnemann School of Medicine

Allan B. Schwartz MD
Professor of Medicine
Section Chief, Hahnemann University
Hospital
MCP Hahnemann School of Medicine

Kumar Sharma MD
Assistant Professor of Medicine
Division of Nephrology
Jefferson Medical College

Michael S. Sherman M.D.
Associate Professor of Medicine
Division of Pulmonary and Critical Care
MCP Hahnemann School of Medicine

Richard L. Spielvogel MD
Professor and Chair,
Department of Dermatology
MCP Hahnemann School of Medicine

Carole E. Thomas MD
Assistant Professor of Neurology
MCP Hahnemann School of Medicine

James Witek M.D.
Assistant Professor of Medicine
MCP Hahnemann School of Medicine

Howard H. Weitz M.D.
Deputy Chairman
Department of Medicine
Jefferson Medical College

Eric T. Wittbrodt, Pharm. D.
Assistant Professor of Clinical
Pharmacology
Philadelphia College of Pharmacy
University of the Sciences in Philadelphia

Preface

In recent years, there has been a virtual explosion of clinical pathways and guidelines relating to treatment of a wide array of common medical conditions. Unfortunately, such pathways and guidelines developed by expert panels may not be widely disseminated or easily locatable at the time of the patient encounter, when on the spot decisions are required. Many of us may be unaware that guidelines even exist for commonly treated conditions. We developed *The Pocket Doctor* as a manual of instantly accessible therapeutic algorithms for common medical conditions based on many of these published clinical guidelines and pathways. Where such pathways may not exist, we have asked our expert authors to devise logical therapeutic strategies based on reliable medical literature as well as their specialized knowledge and experience. Authors have been given the latitude to update published guidelines when, in their opinion, valuable new therapies or drugs have emerged. We have also included a number of helpful tables, which have useful applications in clinical practice.

We have designed this book as a practical guide to patient management. We also believe it will be a valuable teaching aid, as the algorithms present a logical approach to the diagnosis and treatment of a broad range of medical problems. Most of our algorithms and tables have pertinent up-to-date references, which can be used as a further resource. Annotations and added source material, as well as available links to abstracts and full texts of references, will be accessible on our web site, **www.PocketDoctor.com.**

We have had the privilege of working with experts across the country in a broad range of medical fields and wish to thank all of them for their exhaustive efforts in writing and extensively revising the chapters in this book. We would like to thank Jerry Newman, Joy Newman, Lawrence Husick, Teri Deakens RN, Robert Groebel and Niels Buessem for their enthusiastic support and assistance. Special thanks go to our wives, Jennifer and Rebecca, and our children, Rachel, Rebecca, Jeffrey, and Jane, for tolerating and encouraging us during the creation of this project.

Michael S. Sherman, MD
Edward S. Schulman, MD

1a: Periodic Health Examination for the General Population

Screening

Intervention	Age 25-49	Age 50-64	Age ≥ 65
Blood pressure	Q 2 years if last BP < 140/85. Q 1 year if last diastolic was 85-89		
Height and weight	Optimal frequency not defined. Monitor for unintended weight gain/loss and for obesity. Obesity defined as BMI (weight in kg/height in meters) ≥ 27.8 for men and ≥ 27.3 for women		
Total blood cholesterol	Q 5 years (recommendations vary), starting at 35 for men or 45 for women.	Q 5 years (recommendations vary)	Insufficient evidence for routine screening; screen depending on risk.
Fecal occult blood test	For clinical indications		Annual
Sigmoidoscopy	For clinical indications	USPSTF: Insufficient evidence for recommendation ACS: Q 3-5 years ACP: Q 10 years	USPSTF: Insufficient evidence for recommendation ACS: Q 3-5 years ACP: Q 10 years until age 70
Mammogram	USPSTF: Insufficient evidence for recommendation ACS, ACP: Q 1-2 years after age 40	USPSTF: Q 1-2 years ACP, ACS: Annual	USPSTF: Q 1-2 years until age 69 ACP: Annual until age 74
Breast examination	USPSTF: Insufficient evidence for recommendation ACS, ACP: Annual	Annual	USPSTF: Annual until age 70. Screening in older women should be considered on an individual basis.
Pap test	At onset of sexual activity and then Q 3 years	Q 3 years	Q 3 years; consider discontinuing if prior smears are consistently normal
Rubella serology or vaccination history	All women of childbearing potential	Not indicated	Not indicated
Prostate specific antigen (PSA) and digital exam of prostate	For clinical indications	USPSTF: Routine screening is not recommended ACP: Physicians should discuss and individualize decision to screen based on assessment of risk/benefit to the patient (age 50 – 69).	
TSH	For clinical indications	Once (esp females), then as indicated	For clinical indications

Counselling

Intervention	Age 25-49	Age 50-64	Age ≥ 65
Tobacco cessation	Each visit. Prescription of nicotine replacement therapy recommended as adjunct to counselling.		
Assess for problem drinking	All adults and adolescents - careful history and/or standardized questionaire. Pregnant women should be advised to abstain from alcohol during pregnancy. Counsel to avoid alcohol/drug use while driving, swimming, boating, etc.		
Dietary counseling:	Limit to <30% of total calories and saturated fat to < 10 % of total calories. Limit cholesterol to < 300 mg/d. Emphasize foods containing fiber (fruits, whole grains, vegetables), lean meats, fish, poultry without skin, and low fat dairy products.		
Dietary calcium (women)	1,000 mg/day 1,200 -1,500 mg/d if pregnant or nursing	1,000 - 1,500 mg/day	1,000 - 1,500 mg/day

Recommendations are for general population not at high risk. Screening interventions will differ for patients in high risk groups. Except where noted, recommendations are from the Report of the U.S. Preventive Services Task Force (USPSTF). Other organizations may have different recommendations, some of which are noted above. ACP - American College of Physicians. ACS - American Cancer Society.

U.S. Preventive Services Task Force. Guide to clinical preventive services, 2nd ed. Baltimore: William & Wilkins, 1996 (http://text.nlm.nih.gov)

1b: Recommendations for routine vaccinations and post-exposure prophylaxis in adults

Vaccinations

Vaccine	Age 25-49	Age 50-64	Age ≥ 65
Influenza vaccine	Health care providers, residents of chronic care facilities, patients with chronic cardiopulmonary disorders, diabetes, immunosuppression, renal dysfunction, and metabolioic diseases, should also be vaccinated.		All persons
Tetanus vaccine series	All patients who have not received the primary tetanus series. Dose: 0, 2, and 8-14 months.		
Tetanus booster	Optimal frequency not established. Q 15-30 years felt to be adequate. Q 10 years for international travelers.		
Pneumococcal vaccine	Persons at high risk: cardiopulmonary disease, diabetes, asplenia, high exposure, immunocompromise	Persons at high risk: institutionalized patients	All persons
Hepatitis B	All young adults; susceptible adults in high risk groups including health care workers, homosexual men, IV drug users and their sex partners, persons with multiple sex partners, hemodialysis patients, blood product recipients. Dose: 10 or 20 μg (depending on product) IM at 0, 1 and 6 months. Check antibody response in patients with immunodeficiency.		
MMR vaccine	All persons born after 1956 without immunity (no prior vaccination, and no prior infection by history or serology)	Not indicated	Not indicated
Hepatitis A	Travelers to endemic areas, homosexual men, IV drug users, military personnel, at-risk hospital/laboratory workers. Consider in residents and workers in institutions. Dose: 1,440 U at 0 and 6 to 12 months.		
Varicella	Healthy adults with no h/o varicella or prior vaccination and negative serology. Vaccination should be targeted to population at risk: health care workers, family contacts of immunosuppressed patients, day care centers, other institutions		

Post exposure prophylaxis

Exposure	Prophylaxis
Hepatitis A	Immune globulin 0.02 ml/kg IM within 2 weeks of exposure. Indicated for sexual contacts, close household contacts, staff and children at day care centers, staff and patients of custodial institutions, and food handlers exposed to a patient with Hepatitis A.
Hepatitis B	Unvaccinated exposed person: HBsAg + source: Hepatitis B immunoglobulin (HBIG) 0.06 ml/kg IM. Initiate hepatitis B vaccination series within 7 days Unknown source: Initiate hepatitis B vaccination series within 7 days of exposure Previously vaccinated exposed person: Test exposed person for anti HBs. If < 10 SRU by RIA or negative ELISA, HBIG 0.06 ml/kg IM immediately plus HB Vaccine booster or (if vaccine refused) HBIG 0.06 ml/kg IM immediately and repeat at 1 month.
Meningococcus	Rifampin 600 mg BID X 2 days (contraindicated in pregnancy) OR Ofloxacin 400 mg (single dose; safety in pregnancy not established) Indicated for household or day care contacts, direct exposure to oral secretions of patient with meningococcal infection
Tetanus	Clean, minor, uncontaminated wounds: 0.5 ml tetanus toxoid IM if incomplete primary vaccination series or > 10 years from last tetanus booster. Serious and or contaminated wounds: 0.5 ml tetanus toxoid IM if < 5 years from last tetanus booster. Add human tetanus immune globulin if patient has not completed primary series.

U.S. Preventive Services Task Force. Guide to clinical preventive services, 2nd ed. Baltimore: William & Wilkins, 1996(http://text.nlm.nih.gov)

1c: Osteoporosis

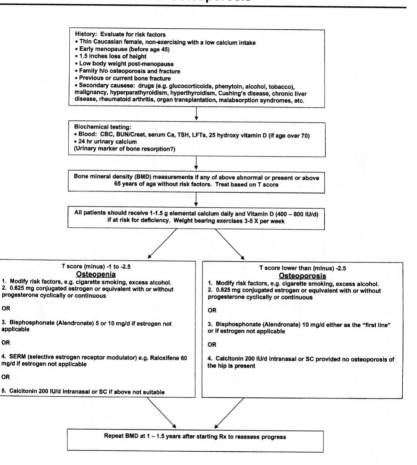

History: Evaluate for risk factors
- Thin Caucasian female, non-exercising with a low calcium intake
- Early menopause (before age 45)
- 1.5 inches loss of height
- Low body weight post-menopause
- Family h/o osteoporosis and fracture
- Previous or current bone fracture
- Secondary causes: drugs (e.g. glucocorticoids, phenytoin, alcohol, tobacco), malignancy, hyperparathyroidism, hyperthyroidism, Cushing's disease, chronic liver disease, rheumatoid arthritis, organ transplantation, malabsorption syndromes, etc.

Biochemical testing:
- Blood: CBC, BUN/Creat, serum Ca, TSH, LFTs, 25 hydroxy vitamin D (if age over 70)
- 24 hr urinary calcium
(Urinary marker of bone resorption?)

Bone mineral density (BMD) measurements if any of above abnormal or present or above 65 years of age without risk factors. Treat based on T score

All patients should receive 1-1.5 g elemental calcium daily and Vitamin D (400 – 800 IU/d) if at risk for deficiency. Weight bearing exercises 3-5 X per week

T score (minus) -1 to -2.5
Osteopenia
1. Modify risk factors, e.g. cigarette smoking, excess alcohol.
2. 0.625 mg conjugated estrogen or equivalent with or without progesterone cyclically or continuous

OR

3. Bisphosphonate (Alendronate) 5 or 10 mg/d if estrogen not applicable

OR

4. SERM (selective estrogen receptor modulator) e.g. Raloxifene 60 mg/d if estrogen not applicable

OR

5. Calcitonin 200 IU/d intranasal or SC if above not suitable

T score lower than (minus) -2.5
Osteoporosis
1. Modify risk factors, e.g. cigarette smoking, excess alcohol.
2. 0.625 mg conjugated estrogen or equivalent with or without progesterone cyclically or continuous

OR

3. Bisphosphonate (Alendronate) 10 mg/d either as the "first line" or if estrogen not applicable

OR

4. Calcitonin 200 IU/d intranasal or SC provided no osteoporosis of the hip is present

Repeat BMD at 1 – 1.5 years after starting Rx to reassess progress

Eastell R. Treatment of postmenopausal osteoporosis. N Engl J Med 338: 736-746, 1998
NOF guidelines. Osteoporosis International 1998 Suppl 4: S1-S88

1d: Prophylaxis for Deep Venous Thrombosis

Procedure or condition	Incidence of DVT	Options for DVT prophylaxis (see *Antithrombotic agents for prophylaxis*)
General surgery	20-25%	Low dose heparin Enoxaparin Dalteparin Extrinsic pneumatic compression (EPC) sleeves or Dextran
Total hip replacement	45-57%	Enoxaparin Danaparoid Warfarin or Adjusted dose heparin May add EPC sleeves as adjuvant Rx
Hip fracture	36-60%	Enoxaparin Danaparoid Warfarin or Adjusted dose heparin May add EPC sleeves as adjuvant Rx
Total knee replacement	40-80%	Enoxaparin or Ardeparin May add EPC sleeves as adjuvant Rx
Craniotomy	18-43%	EPC sleeves Low dose heparin
Acute spinal cord injury	49-72%	Adjusted dose heparin Enoxaparin or Warfarin may be effective (INR 2-3) Low dose heparin plus elastic stockings plus EPC sleeves may have benefit when used together
Spinal cord surgery		EPC sleeves plus low dose heparin EPC sleeves
Gynecologic surgery	Nonmalignancy surgery: Abdominal hysterectomy: 12-15% Vaginal hysterectomy: 6-7% Malignancy surgery: Abdominal hysterectomy: 35%	Low dose heparin Enoxaparin Dalteparin EPC sleeves or Dextran
Urologic surgery	Open prostatectomy: 20-50% TURP: 7-10%	Low dose heparin Enoxaparin Dalteparin or EPC sleeves
General medical patients with clinical risk factors for thromboembolism		Low dose heparin Low molecular weight heparin or EPC sleeves
Myocardial infarction		Heparin (prophylactic low dose or full dose as clinically indicated) Low molecular weight heparin or EPC sleeves when heparin is contraindicated

Warfarin should not be given to pregnant patients.

1e: Anthrombotic agents for deep venous thrombosis prophylaxis

Agent	Dose regimen
Low dose heparin	• Heparin 5,000 U SC Q8 or Q12H. • Begin 2 hours prior to surgery if applicable, continue until discharge
Low molecular weight heparin	Enoxaparin 40 mg SC QD; begin postoperatively for general, urologic, gynecologic surgery. Enoxaparin 30 mg SC Q12h (ASCI, others); begin 12-24 hours postop for ortho surgery (THR, TKR) Danaparoid 750 mg SC Q12h. Begin 1 hr pre-op for ortho surgery (THR) Ardeparin 50 IU/kg SC Q12h. Begin 12 to 24 hours post op for ortho surgery (TKR) Dalteparin 2500 U SC QD. Begin 1 hr prior to surgery

Adjusted Dose Heparin	1. 3500 U SC Q8H postoperatively (0800, 1600, 2400)
	2. Begin adjusting the dose 6 hours following the dose on the evening of surgery. The first adjusted dose will be 2400 hours.
	3. Postop day 1, adjust via dosing schedule below, 6 hours after 0800 hr dose
	4. Adjust every 2nd day 6 hours after the 0800 dose
	5. After 7-10 days begin warfarin (INR 2-3) or maintain the patient on the last total daily adjusted dose of heparin SC Q 12H until discharge.
	6. Schedule for heparin adjustment. You will define the sliding scale based on the top normal PTT of your lab by adding 4 seconds on either side of this value. For example, if the top normal PTT in your lab is 28 seconds, you will aim for a PTT of 28 – 32 seconds and adjust as noted below:
	
	      PTT < 23 seconds ↑ heparin 1,000 U
	      PTT 23-27 seconds ↑ heparin 500 U
	      PTT 28-32 seconds No change
	      PTT 33-37 seconds ↓ heparin 500 U
	      PTT >37 seconds ↓ heparin 1,000 U

Warfarin	• Harris method:
	    10 mg evening prior to surgery
	    5 mg evening of surgery
	    Adjust daily INR to 2-3
	    Continue to discharge
	• Modified method:
	    10 mg the evening of surgery
	    Miss postop day 1
	    Adjust daily INR to 2-3
	    Continue to discharge

Extrinsic pneumatic compression (EPC) sleeves	Place sleeves prior to surgery (if applicable) Sleeves must be worn continuously for 48-72 hours. After 48-72 hours, consider pharmacologic Rx. Patients immobilized >72 hours without prophylaxis must have screening for DVT prior to placing the EPC sleeves
Dextran	500 cc upon initiation of surgery 500 cc postoperatively over 12-18 hours 500 cc daily over 24 hours for 3-5 days (some clinicians prefer to give 10cc/kg during surgery and 7.5 cc/kg daily postoperatively)

ASCI – acute spinal cord injury. THR – total hip replacement. TKR – total knee replacement.

1. Consensus conference. Prevention of venous thrombosis and pulmonary embolism. JAMA 256: 744-749, 1986
2. Merli G, Martinez J. Prophylaxis for deep vein thrombosis and pulmonary embolism in the surgical patient. Med Clin NA 377-397, 1987
3. Goldhaber S, Morpurgo M for the WHO/ISFC Task Force on Pulmonary Embolism. Diagnosis, treatment and prevention of pulmonary embolism. JAMA 268: 1727-1733, 1992
4. Fifth ACCP consensus conference on antithrombotic therapy. Chest 114(suppl): 531S-560S, 1998
5. Merli G. Prophylaxis for deep venous thrombosis and pulmonary embolism in surgery. in Lubin M, Walker HK, and Smith RB III eds, Medical Management of the Surgical Patient, 3rd ed., Lippincott Co., Philadelphia, 1995

2a: Acute Myocardial Infarction

INITIAL ASSESSMENT
- Focused H + P
- Evaluate peripheral perfusion
- ECG- ST elevation> 0.1 mV in at least 2 ant, inf, lat leads; ST depression in ant leads (post. MI)
- Cardiac enzymes (CK-MB, troponins, myoglobin)

IMMEDIATE THERAPY
- IV access
- Cardiac monitoring
- O_2 with continous O_2 monitoring
- ASA 324 mg chew
- Morphine: start 3-5 mg IV, then 2 mg IV q 5' until 16-24 mg or pain relieved
- If tachycardia ± hypertensive: consider beta blocker (see below)

- No ST elevation
- Enzymes negative
See *Management of Unstable Angina*

Negative for MI — Positive for MI

- Consider for Reperfusion Therapy:
Either THROMBOLYSIS* OR ANGIOPLASTY
If neither appropriate/available: Stabilize

THROMBOLYSIS**
- No contraindications*
- MI within 2-6h OR
- MI within 12h with persistent chest pain and ST elevations
- If contraindicated or cardiogenic shock, consider angioplasty

Failure — Success

Consider Angioplasty

ANGIOPLASTY
- Cath lab immediately available (< 1 hour to reperfusion) and/or
- Contraindication to lytic therapy*
- Cardiogenic shock
- Refractory ventricular dysrhythmia
- Large infarct size

Initial Stabilization
Evaluate/ treat complications
of Acute Myocardial Infarction

ADDITIONAL THERAPY / HYPERTENSION
- Relieve pain
- IV NTG: 5-10µg/min initially, increase to 75-100 µg min as BP tolerates
- Beta blockers: e.g. metoprolol 5 mg IV q 5 min. x 3, then 25-50 mg PO q 6 hours
- ACE inhibitors: if no early hypotension: e.g captopril 6.25 mg PO q8 h, increase to 25-50 mg PO q 8 h; OR enalapril 2.5 mg PO q 12h increase to 10-20 mg PO q 12h

HYPOVOLEMIA
- Inferior MI, RV Infarction:
- Rx: rapid IV volume using NS/colloid

SHOCK
- Ventilation/oxygenation
- Immediate primary PTCA
- Hemodynamic monitoring
- Intra-aortic balloon pump
- Pharmacologic support e.g. Dobutamine 2-10 µg/kg/min Dopamine 2-5 µg/kg/min

MECHANICAL PROBLEMS
- Papillary muscle rupture/ dysfunction
- Acute severe mitral regurgitation
- Ventricular septal rupture

Acute Surgical Evaluation / Intervention

DYSRYTHMIA/CONDUCTION DISTURBANCES

Supraventricular tachycardia (SVT)
- DC cardioversion for a fib or SVT if symptoms or hemodynamic instability
- Drugs:
▹ Adenosine: -6 -12 mg IV bolus
Beta blockers:
▹ metoprolol- 5mg. IV q 5 min. X 3 or
▹ propranolol-0.5 - 2 mg IV over 5 min.
Procainamide: 500mg-1gm IV (50mg/min) bolus, then drip at 1-2mg/min

Ventricular tachycardia/fibrillation
- Defibrillate immediately
- Lidocaine 0.5-1mg/kg bolus, infusion 1-4 mg/min.
- Beta blockers IV and oral e.g. metoprolol 5mg IV Q 5 min X 3
- No prophylactic Lidocaine

Bradycardia / AV Block
- Atropine 0.5-1.0 mg if low HR with symptoms , hypotension.
- Stand-by external pacer if risk for:
- complete heart block
- new LBBB with 1°AV block
- new bifasicular block i.e. RBBB + LAH

- Insert temporary transvenous pacemaker if:
Anterior MI with complete heart block;
Inferior MI with heart block and hypoperfusion/symptoms

*CONTRAINDICATIONS to THROMBOLYTIC THERAPY		
ABSOLUTE		**RELATIVE**
Major surgery/trauma < 2 wks	Bleeding diathesis	BP >180/110 on > 2 readings
Aortic dissection	Allergy to agent/prior rxn	Bacterial endocarditis
Active internal bleeding (excluding menses)	CVA known to be hemorrhagic < 12 months	Intraocular bleeding + from diabetic retinopathy
Pericarditis	Pregnancy	CPR < 10 min
Hx of Cerebral tumor/hemorrhage/AVM	History uncontrolled hypertension	Severe renal/liver disease Chronic warfarin therapy
Prolonged traumatic CPR		Stroke/TIA > 12 mos

**Thrombolysis: TPA favored with Anterior MI, age < 75 yr. Dose:- 100 mg IV over 90 minutes given: 15 mg initial IV bolus, then 50 mg IV over 30 min, then 35 mg IV over 60 minutes. OR: Streptokinase-1.5 million U, IV over 30 - 60 minutes
Adjunct RX: Heparin: 80 U/kg IV bolus, then 18U/kg/hr; adjust with PTT (45-70 sec).

1. ACC & AHA Task Force. ACC/AHA Guidelines for management of patients with acute myocardial infarction. J Am Coll Cardiol 28: 1328-1428, 1996
2. The GUSTO Investigators. An international randomized trial comparing four thrombolytic strategies for acute myocardial infarction. N Eng J Med 1993; 329:1615-1622.
3. Anderson, H.V., Willerson, J.E. Thrombolysis in acute myocardial infarction. N Eng J Med 1993;329:703-709.

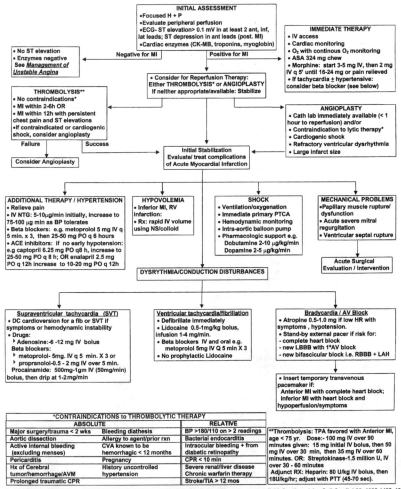

2b: Management of Unstable Angina

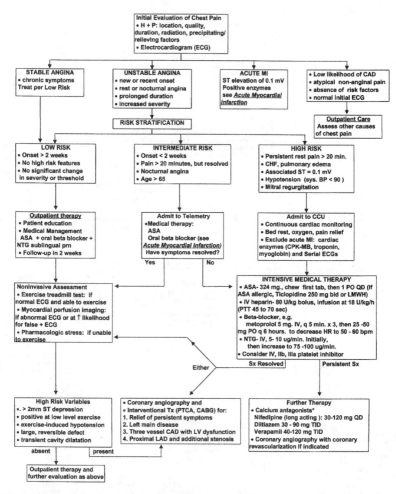

Initial Evaluation of Chest Pain
- H + P: location, quality, duration, radiation, precipitating/relieving factors
- Electrocardiogram (ECG)

STABLE ANGINA
- chronic symptoms Treat per Low Risk

UNSTABLE ANGINA
- new or recent onset
- rest or nocturnal angina
- prolonged duration
- increased severity

ACUTE MI
ST elevation of 0.1 mV
Positive enzymes
see *Acute Myocardial Infarction*

- Low likelihood of CAD
- atypical non-anginal pain
- absence of risk factors
- normal initial ECG

RISK STRATIFICATION

Outpatient Care
Assess other causes of chest pain

LOW RISK
- Onset > 2 weeks
- No high risk features
- No significant change in severity or threshold

INTERMEDIATE RISK
- Onset < 2 weeks
- Pain > 20 minutes, but resolved
- Nocturnal angina
- Age > 65

HIGH RISK
- Persistent rest pain > 20 min.
- CHF, pulmonary edema
- Associated ST = 0.1 mV
- Hypotension (sys. BP < 90)
- Mitral regurgitation

Outpatient therapy
- Patient education
- Medical Management
ASA + oral beta blocker + NTG sublingual prn
- Follow-up in 2 weeks

Admit to Telemetry
- Medical therapy:
ASA
Oral beta blocker (see *Acute Myocardial Infarction*)
Have symptoms resolved?
Yes   No

Admit to CCU
- Continuous cardiac monitoring
- Bed rest, oxygen, pain relief
- Exclude acute MI: cardiac enzymes (CPK-MB, troponin, myoglobin) and Serial ECGs

Noninvasive Assessment
- Exercise treadmill test: if normal ECG and able to exercise
- Myocardial perfusion imaging: if abnormal ECG or at ↑ likelihood for false + ECG
- Pharmacologic stress: if unable to exercise

INTENSIVE MEDICAL THERAPY
- ASA- 324 mg., chew first tab, then 1 PO QD (If ASA allergic, Ticlopidine 250 mg bid or LMWH)
- IV heparin- 80 U/kg bolus, infusion at 18 U/kg/h (PTT 45 to 70 sec)
- Beta-blocker, e.g.
metoprolol 5 mg. IV, q 5 min. x 3, then 25 -50 mg PO q 6 hours. to decrease HR to 50 - 60 bpm
- NTG- IV, 5- 10 ug/min. Initially, then increase to 75 -100 ug/min.
- Consider IV, IIb, IIIa platelet inhibitor

Either   Sx Resolved   Persistent Sx

High Risk Variables
- . > 2mm ST depression
- positive at low level exercise
- exercise-induced hypotension
- large, reversible defect
- transient cavity dilatation
absent

- Coronary angiography and
- Interventional Tx (PTCA, CABG) for:
1. Relief of persistent symptoms
2. Left main disease
3. Three vessel CAD with LV dysfunction
4. Proximal LAD and additional stenosis
present

Further Therapy
- Calcium antagonists*
Nifedipine (long acting): 30-120 mg QD
Diltiazem 30 - 90 mg TID
Verapamil 40-120 mg TID
- Coronary angiography with coronary revascularization if indicated

Outpatient therapy and further evaluation as above

* Calcium antagonists are 2nd line therapy to be used only if symptoms persist despite β-blocker, Nitrates, ASA and heparin. They should be used with extreme caution in patients with LV dysfunction. LMWH – low molecular weight heparin. PTCA –coronary angioplasty

1. Braunwald E, Mark MB, Jones RH, et al. Unstable Angina: Diagnosis and Management. Clinical Practice Guideline Number 10. AHCPR No 94-0602. Rockville, Md., 1994.
2. McClellan JR. Unstable Angina: Prognosis, Noninvasive Risk Assessment and Strategies for Management. Clin Cardiol 1994: 17:229-238
3. Giri S, Waters DD. Pathophysiology and Initial Management of the Acute Coronary Syndromes. Curr Opin Cardiol 1996, 11:394-402.

2c: Congestive Heart Failure

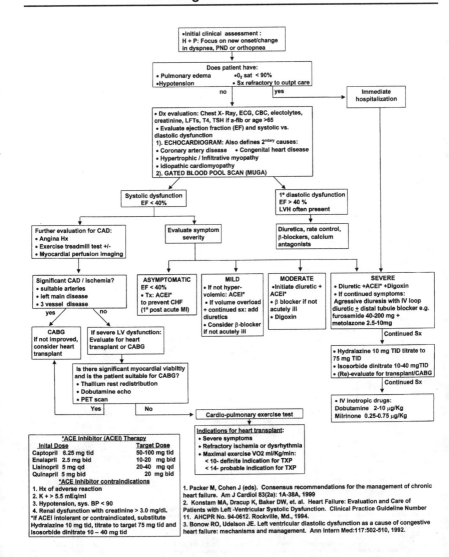

- Initial clinical assessment :
  H + P: Focus on new onset/change
  in dyspnea, PND or orthopnea

Does patient have:
- Pulmonary edema • O₂ sat < 90%
- Hypotension • Sx refractory to outpt care

no → • Dx evaluation: Chest X- Ray, ECG, CBC, electolytes, creatinine, LFTs, T4, TSH if a-fib or age >65
• Evaluate ejection fraction (EF) and systolic vs. diastolic dysfunction
1). ECHOCARDIOGRAM: Also defines 2ndary causes:
  • Coronary artery disease • Congenital heart disease
  • Hypertrophic / Infiltrative myopathy
  • Idiopathic cardiomyopathy
2). GATED BLOOD POOL SCAN (MUGA)

yes → Immediate hospitalization

Systolic dysfunction EF < 40%

1° diastolic dysfunction EF > 40 % LVH often present

Further evaluation for CAD:
- Angina Hx
- Exercise treadmill test +/-
- Myocardial perfusion imaging

Evaluate symptom severity

Diuretics, rate control, β-blockers, calcium antagonists

Significant CAD / ischemia?
- suitable arteries
- left main disease
- 3 vessel disease

yes / no

ASYMPTOMATIC
EF < 40%
- Tx: ACEI*
to prevent CHF
(1° post acute MI)

MILD
- If not hyper-volemic: ACEI*
- If volume overload + continued sx: add diuretics
- Consider β-blocker if not acutely ill

MODERATE
- Initiate diuretic + ACEI*
- β blocker if not acutely ill
- Digoxin

SEVERE
- Diuretic +ACEI* +Digoxin
- If continued symptoms: Agressive diuresis with IV loop diuretic e.g. furosemide 40-200 mg + metolazone 2.5-10mg

CABG
If not improved, consider heart transplant

If severe LV dysfunction: Evaluate for heart transplant or CABG

Is there significant myocardial viability and is the patient suitable for CABG?
- Thallium rest redistribution
- Dobutamine echo
- PET scan

Yes / No

Cardio-pulmonary exercise test

Continued Sx

- Hydralazine 10 mg TID titrate to 75 mg TID
- Isosorbide dinitrate 10-40 mgTID
- (Re)-evaluate for transplant/CABG

Continued Sx

- IV inotropic drugs:
  Dobutamine 2-10 μg/Kg
  Milrinone 0.25-0.75 μg/Kg

Indications for heart transplant:
- Severe symptoms
- Refractory ischemia or dysrhythmia
- Maximal exercise VO2 ml/Kg/min:
  < 10- definite indication for TXP
  < 14- probable indication for TXP

*ACE Inhibitor (ACEI) Therapy	
Inital Dose	**Target Dose**
Captopril 6.25 mg tid	50-100 mg tid
Enalapril 2.5 mg bid	10-20 mg bid
Lisinopril 5 mg qd	20-40 mg qd
Quinapril 5 mg bid	20 mg bid

*ACE inhibitor contraindications
1. Hx of adverse reaction
2. K + > 5.5 mEq/ml
3. Hypotension, sys. BP < 90
4. Renal dysfunction with creatinine > 3.0 mg/dL
*If ACEI intolerant or contraindicated, substitute Hydralazine 10 mg tid, titrate to target 75 mg tid and Isosorbide dinitrate 10 – 40 mg tid

1. Packer M, Cohen J (eds). Consensus recommendations for the management of chronic heart failure. Am J Cardiol 83(2a): 1A-38A, 1999
2. Konstam MA, Dracup K, Baker DW, et. al. Heart Failure: Evaluation and Care of Patients with Left -Ventricular Systolic Dysfunction. Clinical Practice Guideline Number 11. AHCPR No. 94-0612. Rockville, Md., 1994.
3. Bonow RO, Udelson JE. Left ventricular diastolic dysfunction as a cause of congestive heart failure: mechanisms and management. Ann Intern Med:117:502-510, 1992.

2d: Supraventricular Tachycardia

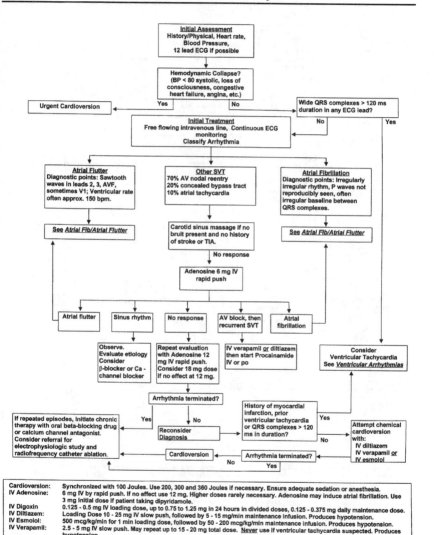

Initial Assessment
History/Physical, Heart rate,
Blood Pressure,
12 lead ECG if possible

Hemodynamic Collapse?
(BP < 80 systolic, loss of
consciousness, congestive
heart failure, angina, etc.)

Yes → **Urgent Cardioversion**

No

**Wide QRS complexes > 120 ms
duration in any ECG lead?**

No

Yes

Initial Treatment
Free flowing intravenous line, Continuous ECG
monitoring
Classify Arrhythmia

Atrial Flutter
Diagnostic points: Sawtooth
waves in leads 2, 3, AVF,
sometimes V1; Ventricular rate
often approx. 150 bpm.

See Atrial Fib/Atrial Flutter

Other SVT
70% AV nodal reentry
20% concealed bypass tract
10% atrial tachycardia

Carotid sinus massage if no
bruit present and no history
of stroke or TIA.

No response

Adenosine 6 mg IV
rapid push

Atrial Fibrillation
Diagnostic points: Irregularly
irregular rhythm, P waves not
reproducibly seen, often
irregular baseline between
QRS complexes.

See Atrial Fib/Atrial Flutter

| Atrial flutter | Sinus rhythm | No response | AV block, then recurrent SVT | Atrial fibrillation |

Observe.
Evaluate etiology
Consider
β-blocker or Ca -
channel blocker

Repeat evaluation
with Adenosine 12
mg IV rapid push.
Consider 18 mg dose
if no effect at 12 mg.

IV verapamil or diltiazem
then start Procainamide
IV or po

Consider
Ventricular Tachycardia
See *Ventricular Arrhythmias*

Arrhythmia terminated?

If repeated episodes, initiate chronic
therapy with oral beta-blocking drug
or calcium channel antagonist.
Consider referral for
electrophysiologic study and
radiofrequency catheter ablation.

Yes

No → Reconsider Diagnosis

History of myocardial
infarction, prior
ventricular tachycardia
or QRS complexes > 120
ms in duration?

Yes

No

Attempt chemical
cardioversion
with:
IV diltiazem
IV verapamil or
IV esmolol

Cardioversion ← No ← **Arrhythmia terminated?** ← Yes

Cardioversion:	Synchronized with 100 Joules. Use 200, 300 and 360 Joules if necessary. Ensure adequate sedation or anesthesia.
IV Adenosine:	6 mg IV by rapid push. If no effect use 12 mg. Higher doses rarely necessary. Adenosine may induce atrial fibrillation. Use 3 mg initial dose if patient taking dipyridamole.
IV Digoxin:	0.125 - 0.5 mg IV loading dose, up to 0.75 to 1.25 mg in 24 hours in divided doses, 0.125 - 0.375 mg daily maintenance dose.
IV Diltiazem:	Loading Dose 10 - 25 mg IV slow push, followed by 5 - 15 mg/min maintenance infusion. Produces hypotension.
IV Esmolol:	500 mcg/kg/min for 1 min loading dose, followed by 50 - 200 mcg/kg/min maintenance infusion. Produces hypotension.
IV Verapamil:	2.5 - 5 mg IV slow push. May repeat up to 15 - 20 mg total dose. Never use if ventricular tachycardia suspected. Produces hypotension.

Adult Advanced Cardiac Life Support. JAMA 1992; 268:2199-2241.

2e: Atrial Fibrillation / Atrial Flutter

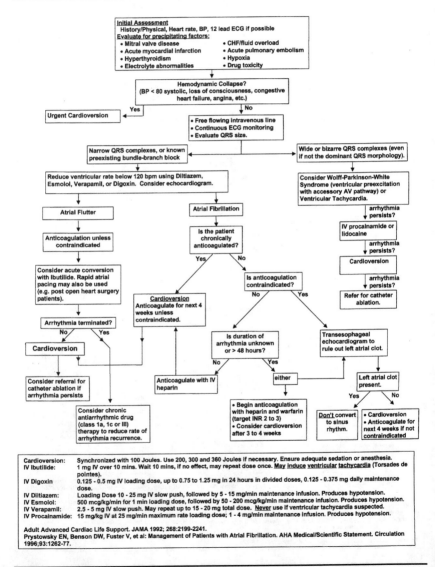

Initial Assessment
History/Physical, Heart rate, BP, 12 lead ECG if possible
Evaluate for precipitating factors:
- Mitral valve disease
- Acute myocardial infarction
- Hyperthyroidism
- Electrolyte abnormalities
- CHF/fluid overload
- Acute pulmonary embolism
- Hypoxia
- Drug toxicity

Hemodynamic Collapse?
(BP < 80 systolic, loss of consciousness, congestive heart failure, angina, etc.)

Yes → **Urgent Cardioversion**

No →
- Free flowing intravenous line
- Continuous ECG monitoring
- Evaluate QRS size.

Narrow QRS complexes, or known preexisting bundle-branch block

Wide or bizarre QRS complexes (even if not the dominant QRS morphology).

Reduce ventricular rate below 120 bpm using Diltiazem, Esmolol, Verapamil, or Digoxin. Consider echocardiogram.

Consider Wolff-Parkinson-White Syndrome (ventricular preexcitation with accessory AV pathway) or Ventricular Tachycardia.

Atrial Flutter

Atrial Fibrillation

arrhythmia persists? → IV procainamide or lidocaine

arrhythmia persists? → Cardioversion

arrhythmia persists? → Refer for catheter ablation.

Anticoagulation unless contraindicated

Is the patient chronically anticoagulated?

Consider acute conversion with Ibutilide. Rapid atrial pacing may also be used (e.g. post open heart surgery patients).

Yes / No

Is anticoagulation contraindicated?

Cardioversion
Anticoagulate for next 4 weeks unless contraindicated.

No / Yes

Arrhythmia terminated?

No / Yes

Cardioversion

Is duration of arrhythmia unknown or > 48 hours?

Transesophageal echocardiogram to rule out left atrial clot.

No / Yes

Consider referral for catheter ablation if arrhythmia persists

Anticoagulate with IV heparin

either

Left atrial clot present.

Yes / No

Consider chronic antiarrhythmic drug (class 1a, 1c or III) therapy to reduce rate of arrhythmia recurrence.

- Begin anticoagulation with heparin and warfarin (target INR 2 to 3)
- Consider cardioversion after 3 to 4 weeks

Don't convert to sinus rhythm.

- Cardioversion
- Anticoagulate for next 4 weeks if not contraindicated

Cardioversion:	Synchronized with 100 Joules. Use 200, 300 and 360 Joules if necessary. Ensure adequate sedation or anesthesia.
IV Ibutilide:	1 mg IV over 10 mins. Wait 10 mins, if no effect, may repeat dose once. **May induce** <u>ventricular tachycardia</u> (Torsades de pointes).
IV Digoxin:	0.125 - 0.5 mg IV loading dose, up to 0.75 to 1.25 mg in 24 hours in divided doses, 0.125 - 0.375 mg daily maintenance dose.
IV Diltiazem:	Loading Dose 10 - 25 mg IV slow push, followed by 5 - 15 mg/min maintenance infusion. Produces hypotension.
IV Esmolol:	500 mcg/kg/min for 1 min loading dose, followed by 50 - 200 mcg/kg/min maintenance infusion. Produces hypotension.
IV Verapamil:	2.5 - 5 mg IV slow push. May repeat up to 15 - 20 mg total dose. **Never** use if ventricular tachycardia suspected.
IV Procainamide:	15 mg/kg IV at 25 mg/min maximum rate loading dose; 1 - 4 mg/min maintenance infusion. Produces hypotension.

Adult Advanced Cardiac Life Support. JAMA 1992; 268:2199-2241.
Prystowsky EN, Benson DW, Fuster V, et al: Management of Patients with Atrial Fibrillation. AHA Medical/Scientific Statement. Circulation 1996;93:1262-77.

2f: AV block

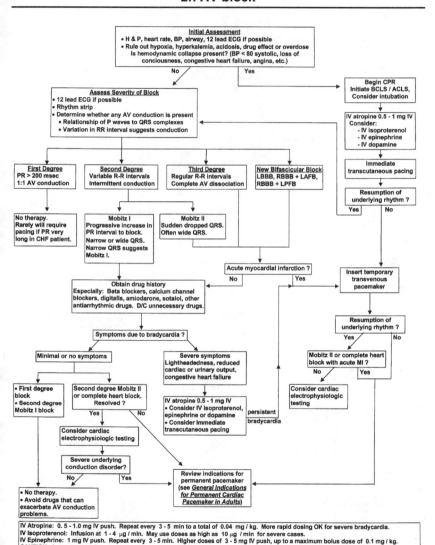

Initial Assessment
- H & P, heart rate, BP, airway, 12 lead ECG if possible
- Rule out hypoxia, hyperkalemia, acidosis, drug effect or overdose
  Is hemodynamic collapse present? (BP < 80 systolic, loss of conciousness, congestive heart failure, angina, etc.)

No → Yes →

Assess Severity of Block
- 12 lead ECG if possible
- Rhythm strip
- Determine whether any AV conduction is present
  - Relationship of P waves to QRS complexes
  - Variation in RR interval suggests conduction

Begin CPR
Initiate BCLS / ACLS,
Consider intubation

IV atropine 0.5 - 1 mg IV
Consider:
- IV isoproterenol
- IV epinephrine
- IV dopamine

Immediate transcutaneous pacing

Resumption of underlying rhythm ?
Yes | No

First Degree
PR > 200 msec
1:1 AV conduction

No therapy. Rarely will require pacing if PR very long in CHF patient.

Second Degree
Variable R-R intervals
Intermittent conduction

Mobitz I
Progressive increase in PR interval to block. Narrow or wide QRS. Narrow QRS suggests Mobitz I.

Third Degree
Regular R-R intervals
Complete AV dissociation

Mobitz II
Sudden dropped QRS. Often wide QRS.

New Bifascicular Block
LBBB, RBBB + LAFB, RBBB + LPFB

Acute myocardial infarction ?
No | Yes

Insert temporary transvenous pacemaker

Obtain drug history
Especially: Beta blockers, calcium channel blockers, digitalis, amiodarone, sotalol, other antiarrhythmic drugs. D/C unnecessary drugs.

Resumption of underlying rhythm ?
Yes | No

Symptoms due to bradycardia ?

Minimal or no symptoms

Severe symptoms
Lightheadedness, reduced cardiac or urinary output, congestive heart failure

Mobitz II or complete heart block with acute MI ?
No | Yes

- First degree block
- Second degree Mobitz I block

Second degree Mobitz II or complete heart block. Resolved ?
Yes | No

IV atropine 0.5 - 1 mg IV
- Consider IV isoproterenol, epinephrine or dopamine
- Consider immediate transcutaneous pacing

persistent bradycardia

Consider cardiac electrophysiologic testing

Consider cardiac electrophysiologic testing

Severe underlying conduction disorder?
No | Yes

Review indications for permanent pacemaker
(see *General Indications for Permanent Cardiac Pacemaker in Adults*)

- No therapy.
- Avoid drugs that can exacerbate AV conduction problems.

IV Atropine: 0.5 - 1.0 mg IV push. Repeat every 3 - 5 min to a total of 0.04 mg / kg. More rapid dosing OK for severe bradycardia.
IV Isoproterenol: Infusion at 1 - 4 µg / min. May use doses as high as 10 µg / min for severe cases.
IV Epinephrine: 1 mg IV push. Repeat every 3 - 5 min. Higher doses of 3 - 5 mg IV push, up to a maximum bolus dose of 0.1 mg / kg.
CAUTION: Isoproterenol & epinephrine may exacerbate tachyarrhythmias, especially SVT, atrial fibrillation, and VT or VF.

Adult Advanced Cardiac Life Support. JAMA 1992; 268: 2199-2241.

2g: Bradycardia

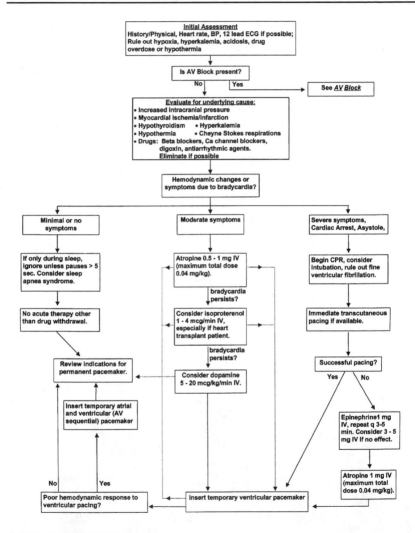

Initial Assessment
History/Physical, Heart rate, BP, 12 lead ECG if possible;
Rule out hypoxia, hyperkalemia, acidosis, drug
overdose or hypothermia

Is AV Block present?

No / Yes → See *AV Block*

Evaluate for underlying cause:
- Increased intracranial pressure
- Myocardial ischemia/infarction
- Hypothyroidism • Hyperkalemia
- Hypothermia • Cheyne Stokes respirations
- Drugs: Beta blockers, Ca channel blockers,
  digoxin, antiarrhythmic agents.
  Eliminate if possible

Hemodynamic changes or
symptoms due to bradycardia?

Minimal or no symptoms

If only during sleep,
ignore unless pauses > 5
sec. Consider sleep
apnea syndrome.

No acute therapy other
than drug withdrawal.

Moderate symptoms

Atropine 0.5 - 1 mg IV
(maximum total dose
0.04 mg/kg).

bradycardia persists?

Consider isoproterenol
1 - 4 mcg/min IV,
especially if heart
transplant patient.

bradycardia persists?

Consider dopamine
5 - 20 mcg/kg/min IV.

Severe symptoms, Cardiac Arrest, Asystole,

Begin CPR, consider
intubation, rule out fine
ventricular fibrillation.

Immediate transcutaneous
pacing if available.

Successful pacing?

Yes / No

Epinephrine1 mg
IV, repeat q 3-5
min. Consider 3 - 5
mg IV if no effect.

Atropine 1 mg IV
(maximum total
dose 0.04 mg/kg).

Review indications for
permanent pacemaker.

Insert temporary atrial
and ventricular (AV
sequential) pacemaker

No / Yes

Poor hemodynamic response to
ventricular pacing?

Insert temporary ventricular pacemaker

Dotted lines indicate acceptable alternatives

Adult Advanced Cardiac Life Support. JAMA 1992; 268:2199-2241

2h: Ventricular Arrhythmias

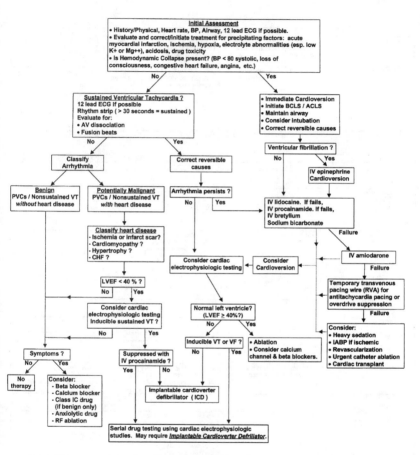

IV epinephrine:	1 mg IV push. May repeat in 3 - 5 min. Maximum bolus is 0.1 mg/kg.
IV lidocaine:	1 - 1.5 mg/kg IV push. Repeat: 0.5 - 0.75 mg/kg IV push q 5 - 10 min to a maximum of 3 mg/kg. Start infusion at 2 - 4 mg/min.
IV procainamide:	17 mg/kg IV at 25 mg / min maximum loading rate. 1 - 4 mg/min maintenance infusion. May cause hypotension.
IV bretylium:	5 - 10 mg/kg IV over 8 - 10 min. Maximum bolus is 30 mg/kg over 24 hours. May cause hypotension.
IV amiodarone:	150 - 300 mg IV over 10 - 20 min; 1 mg/min IV for 6 hours; 0.5 mg/min IV maintenance.
Sodium bicarbonate:	1 mEq/kg IV. Additional doses as required for acidosis.
Cardioversion:	Synchronize for organized VT at 25 - 360 Joules. Asynchronous for VF at 200 - 360 Joules. Use sedation.

Adult Advanced Cardiac Life Support. JAMA 1992; 268: 2199 - 2241.

2i: Antiarrhythmic Drugs

Class Ia

Drug	Dose IV	Dose PO	Therapeutic Level
Quinidine	6 - 10 mg/kg very slow IV infusion as loading dose (at least 1 hour). Generally not recommended as IV therapy.	200 - 600 mg q6 hours immediate release; 200 - 648 mg q8 - 12 hours sustained release.	3 - 6 mcg/ml
Procainamide	15 mg/kg IV at 25 mg/min loading dose, 1 - 5 mg/min maintenance infusion.	250 - 750 mg q4 - 6 hours immediate release; 500 - 1250 mg q6 - 12 hours sustained release	Procainamide 5 - 12 mcg/ml, N-acetylprocainamide 5 - 12 mcg/ml
Disopyramide	N/A	100 - 200 mg q6 hours immediate release; 200 - 400 mg q12 hours sustained release.	3 - 8 mcg/ml

Class Ib

Drug	Dose IV	Dose PO	Therapeutic Level
Lidocaine	1 mg/kg loading dose, 0.5 mg/kg 5-10 min later, followed by 1 - 4 mg/min maintenance infusion.	N/A	2 - 5 mcg/ml
Mexiletine	N/A	150 - 400 mg q8 hours with food	0.5 - 2 mcg/ml
Tocainide	N/A	400 - 600 mg q8-12 hours.	4 - 10 mcg/ml

Class Ic

Drug	Dose IV	Dose PO	Therapeutic Level
Propafenone	N/A	150 - 300 q8 hours.	N/A
Flecainide	N/A	50 - 200 q12 hours.	0.3 - 1.0 mcg/ml.
Moricizine	N/A	200 - 300 mg q8 hours	N/A

Class II

Drug	Dose IV	Dose PO	Therapeutic Level
Propranolol	0.5 - 2.0 mg slow push q2 - 4 hours.	10 - 80 mg q6 hours immediate release; 40 - 160 mg q12 hours or daily sustained release.	N/A
Esmolol	500 mcg/kg/min for 1 minute loading dose, 50 - 200 mcg/kg/min maintenance infusion.	N/A	N/A
Metoprolol	5.0 mg slow push, up to maximum of 15 mg.	25 - 200 mg q12 hours immediate release; 50 - 400 mg daily sustained release.	N/A

Class III

Drug	Dose IV	Dose PO	Therapeutic Level
Bretylium	5 - 10 mg/kg loading dose; 1 - 2 mg/min maintenance infusion.	N/A	N/A
Sotalol	N/A	80 - 240 mg q12 hours	N/A
Ibutilide	1 mg over 10 min, may repeat x1 after additional 10 min. Use less if weight less than 60 kg.	N/A	N/A
Amiodarone	150 mg over 10 min loading dose, followed by 1.0 mg/min for 6 hours then 0.5 mg/min.	800 - 1600 mg loading dose in divided doses for 5 to 14 days, then 600 - 800 mg daily for 2 to 6 weeks, then 200 - 400 mg daily.	Amiodarone 0.8 - 1.5 mcg/ml, Desethylamiodarone similar

Class IV

Drug	Dose IV	Dose PO	Therapeutic Level
Verapamil	2.5 - 5 mg slow push.	40 - 120 mg q8 hours immediate release; 120 - 240 mg daily - q12 hours sustained release.	N/A
Diltiazem	10 - 20 mg slow push loading dose, 5 - 15 mg/min maintenance infusion.	30 - 120 mg q6 - 8 hours immediate release; 120 - 360 mg daily sustained release.	N/A

Miscellaneous

Drug	Dose IV	Dose PO	Therapeutic Level
Adenosine	6 - 18 mg rapid push	N/A	N/A
Digoxin	0.125 - 0.5 mg slow push, up to 0.75 - 1.25 mg / 24 hours	0.125 - 0.375 mg daily	0.5 - 2.0 ng/ml.
Digoxin Antibodies	40 mg (1 vial) for each 0.6 mg of total body store of digoxin. 240 mg typical for adult toxicity except for intentional overdose. See package insert.	N/A	N/A

N/A: not available or not released in the United States as of this writing.

2j: General Indications for Permanent Cardiac Pacemaker Implantation in Adults

General Indications for Permanent Cardiac Pacemaker Implantation in Adults
1. Complete AV block.
2. Second degree AV block, Mobitz 2 or Mobitz I if block intra-His or infra-His.
3. Bilateral bundle branch block after myocardial infarction.
4. Transient advanced AV block with bundle branch block after myocardial infarction.
5. Persistent advanced AV block after myocardial infarction.
6. Bifascicular block with intermittent complete heart block and symptomatic bradycardia.
7. Bifascicular block with Mobitz 2 second degree AV block.
8. Bifascicular block with syncope without other cause identified.
9. Markedly prolonged infra-His conduction (HV interval > 100 ms.)
10. Pacing induced infra-His block.
11. Sinus node dysfunction with symptomatic bradycardia.
12. Sinus node dysfunction with heart rates < 40 bpm as a result of necessary drug therapy.
13. Recurrent syncope due to carotid sinus syndrome with pauses > 3 sec.
14. Congenital Long QT syndrome.
15. For control of supraventricular or ventricular tachycardias uncontrollable by any other means.
16. Hypertrophic cardiomyopathy (evolving new indication)

ACC/AHA Task Force Report: Guidelines for Implantation of Cardiac Pacemakers and Antiarrhythmia Devices. J. Am. Coll. Cardiol 1991; 18:1-13

2k: Indications for Implantable Cardioverter - Defibrillator (ICD) Placement

Indications for Implantable Cardioverter - Defibrillator (ICD) Placement

Class I (General agreement that Implantable Cardioverter - Defibrillators are useful for patient management)

• Cardiac arrest due to VF or VT not due to a transient or reversible cause
• Spontaneous sustained VT
• Syncope of undetermined origin with clinically relevant, hemodynamically significant sustained VT or VF induced at electrophysiological study when drug therapy is ineffective, not tolerated or not preferred
• Nonsustained VT with coronary disease, prior MI, LV dysfunction and inducible VF or sustained VT at electrophysiological study that is not suppressible by a class I antiarrhythmic drug.

Class II (Discretionary : Cardioverter - Defibrillator Implantation is performed, but there is less agreement regarding the usefulness of implantation in these patients.)

• Cardiac arrest presumed to be due to VF when electrophysiological testing is precluded by other medical conditions.
• Severe symptoms attributable to sustained ventricular tachyarrhythmias while awaiting cardiac transplantation
• Familial or inherited conditions with a high risk for life-threatening ventricular arrhythmias such as long QT syndrome or hypertrophic cardiomyopathy
• Nonsustained VT with coronary artery disease, prior MI, LV dysfunction and inducible sustained VT or VF at electrophysiological study
• Recurrent syncope of undetermined etiology in the presence of ventricular dysfunction and inducible ventricular arrhythmias at electrophysiological study when other causes of syncope have been excluded

Class III (General agreement that Implantable Cardioverter - Defibrillators are not indicated)

• Syncope of undetermined cause in a patient without inducible ventricular tachyarrhythmias
• Incessant VT or VF
• VF or VT resulting from arrhythmias amenable to surgical or catheter ablation: for example, atrial arrhythmias associated with the Wolf-Parkinson-White syndrome, right ventricular outflow tract VT, idiopathic left ventricular tachycardia, or fascicular VT.
• Ventricular tachyarrhythmias due to transient or reversible disorder (e.g. acute MI, electrolyte imbalance, drugs, or trauma)
• Significant psychiatric illnesses that may be aggravated by device implantation or may preclude systematic follow-up
• Terminal illnesses with projected life expectancy < 6 months
• Patients with coronary artery disease with LV dysfunction and prolonged QRS duration in the absence of spontaneous or inducible sustained or nonsustained VT who are undergoing coronary bypass surgery
• NYHA class IV drug-refractory congestive heart failure in patients who are not candidates for cardiac transplantation

EP testing = electrophysiologic testing, including induction of VT or VF using programmed ventricular stimulation.
VF = ventricular fibrillation.
VT = ventricular tachycardia.

Adapted from:

Gregoratos G et al. ACC/AHA Guidelines for Implantation of Cardiac Pacemakers and Antiarrhythmia Devices: A report of the American College of Cardiology/American Heart Association Task Force on Practice Guidelines (Committee on Pacemaker Implantation). J Am Coll Cardiol 31: 1175-1209, 1998

Moss AJ, et al. Improved Survival with an Implanted Defibrillator in Patients with Prior Myocardial Infarction, Low Ejection Fraction, and Asymptomatic Non-sustained Ventricular Tachycardia. N Engl J Med 337: 1576-83, 1997

2I: Indications for Cardiac Electrophysiologic Testing

Class I (Indicated by general consensus)

- Symptomatic pts with SND in whom SND has not been clearly established as a cause of symptoms.
- Symptomatic pts with AVB in whom His-Purkinje block is suspected as a cause of AVB.
- Symptomatic pts with AVB or bundle branch block in whom VT is suspected as a cause of symptoms.
- Frequent or poorly tolerated SVT unresponsive to drug therapy, to guide medical treatment or perform catheter ablation.
- Pts with WPW referred for catheter ablation due to life threatening or incapacitating arrhythmias or drug intolerance.
- To guide catheter ablative or surgical techniques for SVT or VT and assess the efficacy of such procedures.
- Sustained or symptomatic wide QRS tachycardias to establish a diagnosis and guide therapy.
- Survivors of cardiac arrest due to tachyarrhythmia not associated with, or greater than 48 hours after, acute myocardial infarction.
- Pts with unexplained syncope and known or suspected heart disease with possible brady- or tachyarrhythmias.
- Documented pulse rate inappropriately rapid (> 150 beats/min) with no ECG documentation of arrhythmia.

Class II (Discretionary)

- Symptomatic pts with SND to exclude other arrhythmias (e.g., VT), to assess anterograde & retrograde conduction and vulnerability to atrial tachyarrhythmias to determine appropriate pacing mode, and to assess response to drug therapy.
- Pts with second or third degree AVB to assess the level of block to guide therapy, and to exclude junctional extrasystoles as a cause of pseudo AVB.
- Symptomatic pts with bundle branch block to assess the level and severity of block to guide therapy.
- SVT pts to assess the effect of antiarrhythmic drug therapy on SN function or AV conduction.
- Pts with accessory pathways to determine the type, number, and characteristics of the bypass tracts and determine the response to drug therapy.
- Asymptomatic pts with WPW with a family history of sudden death; to guide participation in high risk occupations or activities ; or in those having other cardiac surgery to consider surgical ablation of the accessory pathway.
- Risk stratification for pts with a reduced left ventricular ejection fraction, especially due to coronary artery disease, and frequent ventricular ectopy or nonsustained VT, especially with a positive signal averaged ECG, who have an increased risk for sudden death.
- To guide drug therapy in pts with inducible sustained or symptomatic VT.
- Pts with PVCs or nonsustained VT and unexplained syncope or presyncope.
- Pts with unexplained syncope without structural heart disease.
- Pts surviving a cardiac arrest due to bradyarrhythmia.
- Sporadic, significant palpitations that cannot be documented on long-term ECG or event records.
- Identification of proarrhythmic (arrhythmia exacerbating) effects in pts who experience symptoms or sustained VT or cardiac arrest while on antiarrhythmic medications.
- Evaluation of pts undergoing implantation of antiarrhythmic devices, including ICDs, plus re-evaluation when antiarrhythmic drug therapy is changed in such pts.
- Pts with congenital complete AVB and a wide QRS escape rhythm.

Class III (Not indicated)

- Pts with SND or AVB when symptoms are clearly related to the arrhythmia, or when clearly caused by drugs or reversible causes (e.g., inferior myocardial infarction).
- Asymptomatic pts with sinus bradyarrhythmias or sinus pauses during sleep.
- First degree AVB or asymptomatic Mobitz I second degree AVB with a narrow QRS complex.
- Asymptomatic pts with transient AVB associated with sinus slowing, consistent with a vagal mechanism.
- Asymptomatic pts with IVCD, bundle branch block, or bifascicular block.
- Asymptomatic pts with WPW syndrome.
- Pts with supraventricular tachycardia with no evidence of pre-excitation, with sufficient information from surface ECG or monitor to determine appropriate therapy, and who can be easily controlled with vagal maneuvers or medications.
- Pts with congenital long QT syndrome, or those with symptomatic acquired long QT syndrome related to an identifiable cause.
- Asymptomatic pts with PVCs or nonsustained VT with structurally normal hearts.
- Pts with a known cause of syncope.
- Pts with sustained VT or VF due to acute myocardial infarction or to reversible electrolyte / metabolic / toxic causes.

AVB	=	atrioventricular block
ICD	=	implantable cardioverter - defibrillator
IVCD	=	intraventricular conduction delay
Pts	=	patients
PVC	=	premature ventricular complex
SND	=	sinus nodal dysfunction
SVT	=	supraventricular tachycardia
VF	=	ventricular fibrillation
VT	=	ventricular tachycardia
WPW	=	Wolff - Parkinson - White syndrome

ACC / AHA Task Force Report : Guidelines for Clinical Intracardiac Electrophysiologic Studies. J Am Coll Cardiol 1989; 14: 1827-1842.

2m: Recommendations for Prophylaxis of Endocarditis

Endocarditis prophylaxis recommended for:	Endocarditis prophylaxis not recommended for:
• *Prosthetic cardiac valves • *Prior episode of bacterial endocarditis • *Surgical systemic-pulmonary shunts/conduits • *Complex cyanotic congenital heart diseases • Other congenital heart diseases as noted on right • Rheumatic/other acquired valvular dysfunction • Hypertrophic cardiomyopathy • Mitral valve prolapse with mitral regurgitation and/or thickened leaflets (or if confirmation of MR/ thickening not available, with immediate need for the procedure) *high risk patients	• Isolated atrial secundum septal defect • >6 months after repair of ASD, VSD, PDA • Prior coronary artery bypass grafts • Mitral valve prolapse without mitral regurgitation • Cardiac pacemakers • Functional/innocent heart murmurs • Implantable defibrillators • Prior rheumatic fever or Kawasaki's disease without valvular dysfunction

Procedures for which antibiotic prophylaxis is recommended	Procedures for which prophylaxis is not recommended
• Dental procedures likely to cause bleeding/bacteremia Professional cleaning, extractions, periodontal procedures, implants, root canal beyond apex, subgingival surgery, orthodontic bands, intraligamentary injections oral surgery involving teeth or gums • Endoscopic retrograde cholangiography with biliary obstruction • Tonsillectomy/adenoidectomy • Surgery involving GI, biliary, or respiratory tracts • Rigid bronchoscopy • Sclerotherapy of esophageal varices • Esophageal stricture dilatation • Incision and drainage of abscesses • Operations involving infected soft tissue • GU procedures with or without infection: Cystoscopy, urethral dilatation, prostatic surgery • GU procedures only if local infection is present: urethral catheterization, urinary tract surgery, vaginal delivery	• Dental procedures unlikely to cause bleeding: Restorative dentistry (fillings), orthodontic adjustments, local oral anesthetic injection (except intraligamentary), intracanal endodontic treatment, placement of rubber dams, post-op suture removal, oral impressions, fluoride treatments, oral X-rays, loss of primary teeth, placement of removable orthodontic or prosthodontic appliances • Tympanostomy tube insertion • Endotracheal intubation • Flexible bronchoscopy (with or without biopsy)[†] • Cardiac catheterization • GI endoscopy (with or without biopsy) [†] • Ceasarean section • Transesophageal echocardiography • GU procedures in the absence of infection: urethral catheterization, D & C, vaginal delivery[†], therapeutic abortion, sterilization procedures, vaginal hysterectomy[†] and IUD insertion/removal • Incision and biopsy of surgically scrubbed skin • Cardiac catheterization/angioplasty/pacemaker/ defibrillators or stent implantation • Circumcision
	† optional in high risk patients

Current Recommendations for Endocarditis Prophylaxis

Indication	Regimen
Dental, oral, respiratory tract or esophageal procedures	• Amoxicillin 2.0 g po 1 hr pre-procedure OR If penicillin allergic (choose one regimen)[‡]: • Clindamycin 600 mg po 1 hr pre-procedure OR • Azithromycin 500 mg po 1 hr pre-procedure OR • Clarithromycin 500 mg po 1 hr pre-procedure OR
Dental, oral, or respiratory tract or esophageal procedures; patients NPO	• Ampicillin 2.0 g 30' pre-procedure IV or IM If penicillin allergic: • Clindamycin 600 mg IV within 30 minutes pre-procedure
Genitourinary and non esophageal gastrointestinal procedures: High risk patients	• Ampicillin 2.0 g IV or IM plus gentamicin 1.5 mg/kg (max 120 mg) 30' pre-procedure, then either amoxicillin 1 g po 6 hrs later or ampicillin 1 g IV 6 h later If penicillin allergic: • Vancomycin 1.0g IV given over 1-2 h, plus gentamicin 1.5 mg/kg (max 120 mg), complete infusion within 30 minutes of starting the procedure
Genitourinary and non esophageal gastrointestinal procedures: Moderate risk patients	• Amoxicillin 2.0 g po 1 hr pre-procedure OR • Ampicillin 2.0 g 30' pre-procedure IV or IM If penicillin allergic: • Vancomycin 1.0g IV 1 hr pre-procedure given over 1 hr, complete within 30 minutes of starting the procedure
‡ Cephalosporin recommendations are not listed because they should not be used in patients with immediate-type hyper-sensitivity reactions to penicillins	

Abbreviations: ASD - atrial septal defect. VSD - ventricular septal defect. PDA - patent ductus arteriosus. D & C - dilation and curettage. IUD - intrauterine device. AHA - American Heart Association.
Tables list those selected procedures and conditions listed in references but are not all-inclusive. Vancomycin and gentamicin should be adjusted for renal impairment

Dajani AS, et al. Prevention of bacterial endocarditis. Recommendations by the American Heart Association. JAMA 277: 1794-1801, 1997 and 264:2919, 1990
Simmons NA. Recommendations for endocarditis prophylaxis. J Antimicrob Chemother 31:437, 1993

2n: Therapy for Infectious Endocarditis

Empiric Therapy for Infective Endocarditis (cultures pending)

Clinical situation	Likely organisms	Antibiotic regimen
Native valve endocarditis	Viridans streptococci Staphylococcus aureus Enterococci	Vancomycin 1 gm IV q12h + Gentamicin 3 mg/kg/d
Early prosthetic valve endocarditis (<2 mos)	Staphylococcus epidermidis Staphylococcus aureus Enterobacteriaciae Diptheroids	Vancomycin 1 gm IV q12h + Gentamicin 3 mg/kg/d +/- Rifampin 600 mg p.o. qd
Late prosthetic valve endocarditis (> 2 mos)	Viridans streptococci Staphylococcus epidermidis Staphylococcus aureus Enterococci	Vancomycin 1 gm IV q12h + Gentamicin 3 mg/kg/d +/- Rifampin 600 mg p.o. qd

Indications for Surgery in Infective Endocarditis

Indications for urgent surgery	Relative indications for surgery
• Refractory heart failure • Persistent bacteremia • Fungal endocarditis • No effective antimicrobial agent available • Prosthetic valve obstruction • Unstable prosthesis	• Nonstreptococcal endocarditis • Relapse • Intracardiac extension of infection • 2 or more systemic emboli • Echocardiogram: -Vegetations -Mitral valve preclosure • Early prosthetic valve endocarditis • Periprosthetic valve leak

Specific Therapy for Native Valve Endocarditis

Organism	Antibiotic regimen	Duration	Comments
Viridans streptococci or Streptococcus bovis (MIC < 0.1 ug/ml PenG)	Penicillin G 2-3 MU IV q4h OR Ceftriaxone 2 g IV qd OR Penicillin G 2-3 MU IV q4h + Gentamicin 3 mg/kg/d OR Vancomycin 1 gm IV q12h	4 weeks 4 weeks 2 weeks 2 weeks 4 weeks	2-week regimen only if no extracardiac foci of infection or intracardiac abscesses. Vancomycin used for patients allergic to β-lactam antibiotics.
Viridans streptococci or Streptococcus bovis (MIC > 0.1 and < 0.5 ug/ml PenG)	Penicillin G 3 MU IV q4h + Gentamicin 3 mg/kg/d OR Vancomycin 1 gm IV q12h	4 weeks 2 weeks 4 weeks	Vancomycin used for patients allergic to β-lactam antibiotics.
Viridans streptococci (MIC > 0.5 ug/ml PenG) Enterococci Nutritionally variant viridans streptococci	Penicillin G 3-5 MU IV q4h + Gentamicin 3 mg/kg/d OR Ampicillin 2 gm IV q4h + Gentamicin 3 mg/kg/d OR Vancomycin 1 gm IV q12h + Gentamicin 3 mg/kg/d	4-6 weeks 4-6 weeks 4-6 weeks 4-6 weeks 4-6 weeks 4-6 weeks	Treatment of enterococci dependent on susceptibilities. Vancomycin used for patients allergic to β-lactam antibiotics or for penicillin-resistant enterococci.
Methicillin-susceptible staphylococcus aureus	Nafcillin or oxacillin 2 gm IV q4h + Gentamicin 3 mg/kg/d (optional) OR Cefazolin 2 gm IV q8h + Gentamicin 3 mg/kg/d (optional) OR Vancomycin 1 gm IV q12h	4-6 weeks 3-5 days 4-6 weeks 3-5 days 4-6 weeks	Aminoglycosides expedite clearance of bacteremia but no proven benefit in clinical outcome. Vancomycine used for patients allergic to β-lactam antibiotics.
Methicillin-resistant staph aureus	Vancomycin 1 gm IV q12h	4-6 weeks	

Specific Therapy for Prosthetic Valve Endocarditis

Organism	Antibiotic regimen	Duration	Comments
Viridans streptococci or Streptococcus bovis (MIC < 0.1 ug/ml PenG)	Penicillin G 3-5 MU IV q4h + Gentamicin 3 mg/kg/d OR Vancomycin 1 gm IV q12h + Gentamicin 3 mg/kg/d	4-6 weeks 2 weeks 4-6 weeks 2 weeks	Vancomycin for patients allergic to β-lactam antibiotics.
Viridans streptococci or Streptococcus bovis (MIC > 0.1 ug/ml PenG) Enterococci Nutritionally variant viridans streptococci	Penicillin G 3-5 MU IV q4h + Gentamicin 3 mg/kg/d OR Ampicillin 2 gm IV q4h + Gentamicin 3 mg/kg/d	6-8 weeks 6-8 weeks 6-8 weeks 6-8 weeks	Vancomycin 1 gm IV q12h can be substituted for penicillin or ampicillin in patients allergic to β-lactam antibiotics or those with penicillin-resistant enterococci.
Methicillin-susceptible staphylococcus aureus	Nafcillin or oxacillin 2 gm IV q4h + Rifampin 600 mg p.o. qd + Gentamicin 3 mg/kg/d	6-8 weeks 6-8 weeks 2 weeks	Cefazolin 2 gm IV q8h substituted for nafcillin in patients with penicillin allergy. Vancomycin 1 gm IV q12h allergic to β-lactam antibiotics..
Methicillin-resistant staphylococcus aureus Coagulase-negative staphylococci	Vancomycin 1 gm IV q12h + Rifampin 600 mg p.o. qd + Gentamicin 3 mg/kg/d	6-8 weeks 6-8 weeks 2 weeks	Rifampin and gentamicin used in methicillin-resistant staphylococcus aureus infection only if organism susceptible.

Wilson WR, et.al. Antibiotic Treatment of Adults with Infective Endocarditis due to Streptococci, Enterococci, Staphylococci, and HACEK Microorganisms. JAMA 274:1706, 1995

Alsip SG, et. al. Indications for Cardiac Surgery in Patients with Active Infectious Endocarditis. Amer J Med 78:138, 1985

2o: Treatment of Hypercholesterolemia

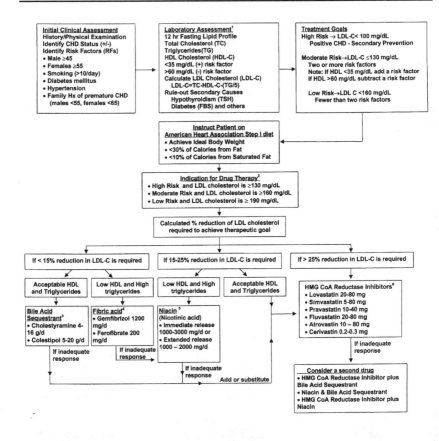

Initial Clinical Assessment
History/Physical Examination
Identify CHD Status (+/-)
Identify Risk Factors (RFs)
- Male ≥45
- Females ≥55
- Smoking (>10/day)
- Diabetes mellitus
- Hypertension
- Family Hx of premature CHD (males <55, females <65)

Laboratory Assessment[1]
12 hr Fasting Lipid Profile
Total Cholesterol (TC)
Triglycerides(TG)
HDL Cholesterol (HDL-C)
<35 mg/dL (+) risk factor
>60 mg/dL (-) risk factor
Calculate LDL Cholesterol (LDL-C)
   LDL-C=TC-HDL-C-(TG/5)
Rule-out Secondary Causes
   Hypothyroidism (TSH)
   Diabetes (FBS) and others

Treatment Goals
High Risk → LDL-C< 100 mg/dL
   Positive CHD - Secondary Prevention

Moderate Risk→LDL-C ≤130 mg/dL
   Two or more risk factors
   Note: If HDL <35 mg/dL add a risk factor
   If HDL >60 mg/dL subtract a risk factor

Low Risk→LDL C <160 mg/dL
   Fewer than two risk factors

Instruct Patient on
American Heart Association Step I diet
- Achieve Ideal Body Weight
- <30% of Calories from Fat
- <10% of Calories from Saturated Fat

Indication for Drug Therapy[2]
- High Risk and LDL cholesterol is ≥130 mg/dL
- Moderate Risk and LDL cholesterol is ≥160 mg/dL
- Low Risk and LDL cholesterol is ≥ 190 mg/dL

Calculated % reduction of LDL cholesterol required to achieve therapeutic goal

If < 15% reduction in LDL-C is required

Acceptable HDL and Triglycerides

Bile Acid Sequestrant[3]
- Cholestyramine 4-16 g/d
- Colestipol 5-20 g/d
If inadequate response

Low HDL and High triglycerides

Fibric acid[4]
- Gemfibrizol 1200 mg/d
- Ferofibrate 200 mg/d
If inadequate response

If 15-25% reduction in LDL-C is required

Low HDL and High triglycerides

Niacin[5]
(Nicotinic acid)
- Immediate release 1000-3000 mg/d or
- Extended release 1000 – 2000 mg/d
If inadequate response
Add or substitute

Acceptable HDL and Triglycerides

If > 25% reduction in LDL-C is required

HMG CoA Reductase Inhibitors[6]
- Lovastatin 20-80 mg
- Simvastatin 5-80 mg
- Pravastatin 10-40 mg
- Fluvastatin 20-80 mg
- Atrovastin 10 – 80 mg
- Cerivastatin 0.2-0.3 mg
If inadequate response

Consider a second drug
- HMG CoA Reductase Inhibitor plus Bile Acid Sequestrant
- Niacin & Bile Acid Sequestrant
- HMG CoA Reductase Inhibitor plus Niacin

1. Ideally 2 measurements 2-6 weeks apart, but not during or in a recovery phase of an acute medical event. LDL-C should be calculated only if triglycerides are ≤ 400 mg/dL..
2. Young men and pre-menopausal women are usually at low risk for CHD unless they have multiple other risk factors (Diabetes Mellitus or family history of premature CHD) or very high LDL-C (≥ 220 mg/dL). In pre-menopausal women not at high risk, drug therapy for high cholesterol levels should generally be delayed.
3. Good efficacy and safety record and can be used in pre-menopausal women but only 10-30% LDL-C reduction.
4. Effective in lowering triglycerides and raising HDL, but minimal effect on LDL-C (10-15% reduction).
5. Lowers triglycerides and LDL-C (10-25% reduction) and raises HDL, but bothersome side effects of flushing, hyperglycemia, pruritis, hyperuricemia, and dose-related hepatotoxicity.
6. Highly effective (20-40% reduction of LDL-C), but long term safety not established and generally not recommended for use in women of childbearing potential.

CHD: Coronary heart disease.

3a: Management of Acute Pulmonary Thromboembolism

Determine clinical suspicion based on:
- History: Sudden onset dyspnea, syncope, substernal chest pain. If pleuritic pain, hemoptysis, likely infarction.
- Physical exam: Tachycardia, tachypnea. Massive PE: RV S3. Pleural rub suggests infarction.
- Laboratories: ↓PO2, ↓PCO2, widened A-a gradient. Normal A-a gradient with PCO2 > 36 rules out PE. CXR often normal or nonspecific; may see infiltrate, effusion with infarction.

Clinical Suspicion

Low → **Consider anticoagulation**

Intermediate or High → **Start anticoagulation if no absolute contraindication**

Either:
- **D/US** — Positive → **Treat***; Negative → **Follow and repeat X 3 over 5-15 days**
- **Ventilation/ Perfusion scan (% with PE)**

Either:
- **D/US** — Negative; Positive → **Treat***

From V/Q scan:

| Normal scan (<1%) | Low Probability (15 – 30%) | Intermediate Probability (>30%) | High Probability (≥ 85%) |

- Normal scan (<1%) → **Follow**
- Low Probability → **Clinical suspicion**: Low (<5%) → **Follow**; High/intermediate → **Serial D/US**
- Intermediate Probability → **Is cardiovascular disease present?**: No → **Angiogram or serial D/US**; Yes (≥15%) → **Angiogram or serial D/US**
- High Probability → **Prior PE or high clinical suspicion?**: No (<75%) → **Angiogram or serial D/US**; Yes (>90%) → **Treat***

Serial D/US: Positive → **Treat***; Negative (<3%) → **Follow**

Angiogram or serial D/US: Negative → **Follow**; Positive → **Treat***

Indications for inferior vena cava filter:
- PE with contraindication to, or complication from, anticoagulation
- Massive PE in a patient in whom a subsequent PE might be fatal
- Consider in high risk patients with: chronic pulmonary hypertension, pre-op pulmonary embolectomy, severe spinal, head, pelvic trauma, "free floating" thrombus
- Recurrent pulmonary embolism despite adequate anticoagulation
- Venogram-documented DVT with contraindication to heparin

D/US: Duplex ultrasound. PE: pulmonary embolism. PE likelihood is indicated in parenthesis (Kelly et al).
*Treat:
If hemodynamically stable: Heparin 5,000 – 10,000U bolus then 1,300 U/h or 80U/kg bolus then 18 U/kg/h. ✓aPPT 6 hr after bolus or dosage change. Start warfarin within 24 h of dx and overlap with heparin > 5 days.
If hemodynamically unstable ± RV hypokinesis on echocardiogram: Consider thrombolytic therapy if no contraindications. Three approved regimens: 1: Streptokinase: Load 250,000 IU X 30', then 100,000 IU/h X 24h. 2: Urokinase Load 4,400 IU/kg X 10', then 4,400 IU/kg/h x 12-24 h. 3: rt-PA: 100 mg continuous peripheral infusion over 2 h. No need to follow aPTT with infusion, but check at end and q4h prn until aPTT <80sec, then start heparin without bolus at 18 U/kg/h or 1,300 U/h.
If anticoagulation contraindicated: place inferior vena cava filter

Kelley MA et al. Diagnosing pulmonary embolism: New facts and strategies. Ann Intern Med 114: 300, 1991
Rosenow EC. Venous and pulmonary thromboembolism: An algorithmic approach to diagnosis and management. Mayo Clin Proc: 70: 45, 1995
Goldhaber SZ. Contemporary pulmonary embolism thrombolysis. Chest 107: 45S, 1995
Litin SC and Gastineau DA. Current consempts in anticoagulant therapy. Mayo Clin Proc 70: 266, 1995
Becker DM et al. Inferior vena cava filters: Indications, safety, effectiveness. Arch Int Med 152: 1985, 1992

3b: Acute Exacerbation of Asthma

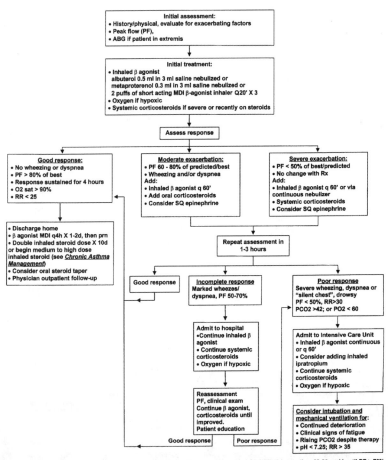

Initial assessment:
- History/physical, evaluate for exacerbating factors
- Peak flow (PF),
- ABG if patient in extremis

Initial treatment:
- Inhaled β agonist
  albuterol 0.5 ml in 3 ml saline nebulized or
  metaproterenol 0.3 ml in 3 ml saline nebulized or
  2 puffs of short acting MDI β-agonist inhaler Q20' X 3
- Oxygen if hypoxic
- Systemic corticosteroids if severe or recently on steroids

Assess response

Good response:
- No wheezing or dyspnea
- PF > 80% of best
- Response sustained for 4 hours
- O2 sat > 90%
- RR < 25

Moderate exacerbation:
- PF 60 - 80% of best/predicted
- Wheezing and/or dyspnea
Add:
- Inhaled β agonist q 60'
- Add oral corticosteroids
- Consider SQ epinephrine

Severe exacerbation:
- PF < 50% of best/predicted
- No change with Rx
Add:
- Inhaled β agonist q 60' or via continuous nebulizer
- Systemic corticosteroids
- Consider SQ epinephrine

- Discharge home
- β agonist MDI q4h X 1-2d, then prn
- Double inhaled steroid dose X 10d or begin medium to high dose inhaled steroid (see *Chronic Asthma Management*)
- Consider oral steroid taper
- Physician outpatient follow-up

Repeat assessment in 1-3 hours

Good response

Incomplete response
Marked wheezes/ dyspnea, PF 50-70%

Poor response
Severe wheezing, dyspnea or "silent chest", drowsy
PF < 50%, RR>30
PCO2 >42; or PO2 < 60

Admit to hospital
- Continue inhaled β agonist
- Continue systemic corticosteroids
- Oxygen if hypoxic

Admit to Intensive Care Unit
- Inhaled β agonist continuous or q 60'
- Consider adding inhaled ipratropium
- Continue systemic corticosteroids
- Oxygen if hypoxic

Reassessment
PF, clinical exam
Continue β agonist, corticosteroids until improved.
Patient education

Consider intubation and mechanical ventilation for:
- Continued deterioration
- Clinical signs of fatigue
- Rising PCO2 despite therapy
- pH < 7.25; RR > 35

Good response   Poor response

- Corticosteroids: Recommended minimum dose - methylprednisolone 120-180 mg/day divided Q6-8H X 48 hours, then 60-80 mg/d until PF ≥ 70% of personal best or predicted
- Epinephrine dose: 0.3 mg of 1:1,000 dilution Q 20' X 3 doses
- Continuous β agonist: Withdraw 16 ml normal saline from 100ml bag; replace with 16 ml albuterol solution; run at 12.5 ml/min into nebulizer = 2 ml albuterol/hour
- Inhaled ipratropium: Ipratropium bromide 3-6 puffs MDI Q4-6H or nebulize 0.5 mg in 3 cc saline Q6H;

Guidelines for the diagnosis and management of asthma, NIH publication No. 97-4051, 1997
International consensus report on diagnosis and treatment of asthma; NIH Publication No. 92-3091, 1992
Guidelines for the diagnosis and management of asthma, NIH Publication No. 91-3042, 1991
Manthous CA. Management of severe exacerbations of asthma. Am J Med 99:298; 1995

3c: Chronic Asthma Management

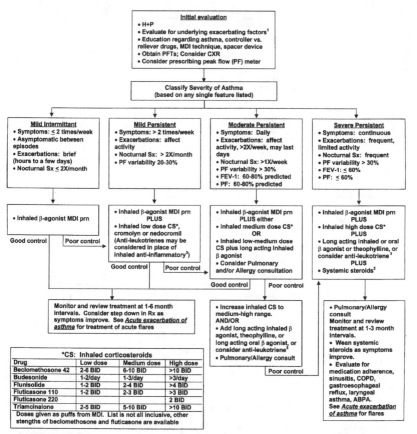

Initial evaluation
- H+P
- Evaluate for underlying exacerbating factors[1]
- Education regarding asthma, controller vs. reliever drugs, MDI technique, spacer device
- Obtain PFTs; Consider CXR
- Consider prescribing peak flow (PF) meter

Classify Severity of Asthma
(based on any single feature listed)

Mild Intermittent
- Symptoms: ≤ 2 times/week
- Asymptomatic between episodes
- Exacerbations: brief (hours to a few days)
- Nocturnal Sx ≤ 2X/month

Mild Persistent
- Symptoms: > 2 times/week
- Exacerbations: affect activity
- Nocturnal Sx: > 2X/month
- PF variability 20-30%

Moderate Persistent
- Symptoms: Daily
- Exacerbations: affect activity, >2X/week, may last days
- Nocturnal Sx: >1X/week
- PF variability > 30%
- FEV-1: 60-80% predicted
- PF: 60-80% predicted

Severe Persistent
- Symptoms: continuous
- Exacerbations: frequent, limited activity
- Nocturnal Sx: frequent
- PF variability > 30%
- FEV-1: ≤ 60%
- PF: ≤ 60%

- Inhaled β-agonist MDI prn

Good control | Poor control

- Inhaled β-agonist MDI prn PLUS
- Inhaled low dose CS*, cromolyn or nedocromil (Anti-leukotrienes may be considered in place of inhaled anti-inflammatory[3])

Good control | Poor control

- Inhaled β-agonist MDI prn PLUS either
- Inhaled medium dose CS* OR
- Inhaled low-medium dose CS plus long acting inhaled β agonist
- Consider Pulmonary and/or Allergy consultation

Good control | Poor control

- Inhaled β-agonist MDI prn PLUS
- Inhaled high dose CS* PLUS
- Long acting inhaled or oral β agonist or theophylline, or consider anti-leukotriene[3] PLUS
- Systemic steroids[2]

Monitor and review treatment at 1-6 month intervals. Consider step down in Rx as symptoms improve. See *Acute exacerbation of asthma* for treatment of acute flares

- Increase inhaled CS to medium-high range. AND/OR
- Add long acting inhaled β agonist, theophylline, or long acting oral β agonist, or consider anti-leukotriene[3]
- Pulmonary/Allergy consult

Poor control

- Pulmonary/Allergy consult Monitor and review treatment at 1-3 month intervals.
- Wean systemic steroids as symptoms improve.
- Evaluate for medication adherence, sinusitis, COPD, gastroesophageal reflux, laryngeal asthma, ABPA. See *Acute exacerbation of asthma* for flares

*CS: Inhaled corticosteroids			
Drug	Low dose	Medium dose	High dose
Beclomethosone 42	2-6 BID	6-10 BID	>10 BID
Budesonide	1-2/day	1-3/day	>3/day
Flunisolide	1-2 BID	2-4 BID	>4 BID
Fluticasone 110	1-2 BID	2-3 BID	>3 BID
Fluticasone 220			2 BID
Triamcinalone	2-5 BID	5-10 BID	>10 BID

Doses given as puffs from MDI. List is not all inclusive, other stengths of beclomethosone and fluticasone are available

1. Exacerbating/risk factors: β blockers, sinusitis, specific allergy (e.g. pets, dust mite, cockroach, mold spores, seasonal), gastro-esophageal reflux, exercise, cold air, aspirin/NSAIDs
2. Prednisone, methylprednisolone or prednisolone, 7.5-60 mg/d, use minimum effective dose. Alternate day therapy preferred for chronic management. Steroid dependent asthmatics should be evaluated by a Pulmonary and/or Allergy specialist
3. The role of anti-leukotriene agents is not clearly defined at publication. Montelukast 10 mg qd, Zafirlukast 20 mg bid, Zileuton 600 mg qid

β-agonist: Albuterol, albuterol HFA, bitolterol, pirbuterol, or terbutraline MDI inhaler, 2 puffs, or albuterol rotocap 1-2 capsules or albuterol solution 1.25-5 mg in 2-3 ml saline. β agonists may be administered Q4-6H prn. Increasing use indicates "poor control".
Long acting β agonist: Inhaled salmeterol 2 puffs BID; oral sustained release albuterol 4-8 mg Q12H
Theophylline: 300-800 mg/day, use sustained release compound and aim for level of 8-12mcg/ml
ABPA: Allergic Broncho-Pulmonary Aspergillosis

Guidelines for the diagnosis and management of asthma, NIH publication No. 97-4051, 1997
International consensus report on diagnosis and treatment of asthma; NIH Publication No. 92-3091, 1992
Guidelines for the diagnosis and management of asthma, NIH Publication No. 91-3042, 1991

3d: Management of Chronic Obstructive Pulmonary Disease

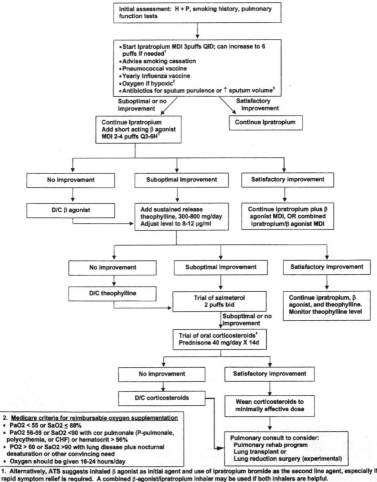

Initial assessment: H + P, smoking history, pulmonary function tests

- Start Ipratropium MDI 3puffs QID; can increase to 6 puffs if needed[1]
- Advise smoking cessation
- Pneumococcal vaccine
- Yearly influenza vaccine
- Oxygen if hypoxic[2]
- Antibiotics for sputum purulence or ↑ sputum volume[3]

Suboptimal or no improvement

Satisfactory improvement

Continue Ipratropium
Add short acting β agonist MDI 2-4 puffs Q3-6H[1]

Continue Ipratropium

No improvement → D/C β agonist

Suboptimal improvement → Add sustained release theophylline, 300-800 mg/day. Adjust level to 8-12 µg/ml

Satisfactory improvement → Continue ipratropium plus β agonist MDI, OR combined ipratropium/β agonist MDI

No improvement → D/C theophylline

Suboptimal improvement → Trial of salmeterol 2 puffs bid

Satisfactory improvement → Continue ipratropium, β agonist, and theophylline. Monitor theophylline level

Suboptimal or no improvement

Trial of oral corticosteroids[4]
Prednisone 40 mg/day X 14d

No improvement → D/C corticosteroids

Satisfactory improvement → Wean corticosteroids to minimally effective dose

2. <u>Medicare criteria for reimbursable oxygen supplementation</u>
- PaO2 < 55 or SaO2 ≤ 88%
- PaO2 56-59 or SaO2 <90 with cor pulmonale (P-pulmonale, polycythemia, or CHF) or hematocrit > 56%
- PO2 > 60 or SaO2 >90 with lung disease plus nocturnal desaturation or other convincing need
- Oxygen should be given 16-24 hours/day

Pulmonary consult to consider:
Pulmonary rehab program
Lung transplant or
Lung reduction surgery (experimental)

1. Alternatively, ATS suggests inhaled β agonist as initial agent and use of ipratropium bromide as the second line agent, especially if rapid symptom relief is required. A combined β-agonist/ipratropium inhaler may be used if both inhalers are helpful.
3. 7 days of broad spectrum po agent e.g.: doxycycline 100 mg bid, trimethoprim sulfasoxazole 1 DS BID, amoxicillin/clavulinic acid 500 mg bid, 2nd generation cephalosporin, clarithromycin 250-500 mg bid, or azithromycin 500 mg on day 1 followed by 250 mg qd for 4 days
4. Inhaled steroids are recommended by some experts; benefit is not fully established. Oral sustained release albuterol may also benefit.

American Thoracic Society. Standards for the diagnosis and care of patients with chronic obstructive lung disease. Am J Crit Care Med 152:S77-S120, 1995
Ferguson GT, Cherniack RM. Management of chronic obstructive pulmonary disease. N Engl J Med 328: 1017, 1993
Murphy TF, Sethi S. Bacterial infection in chronic obstructive pulmonary disease. Am Rev Resp Dis 146: 1067; 1992

3e: Chronic Obstructive Pulmonary Disease - Acute Respiratory Failure

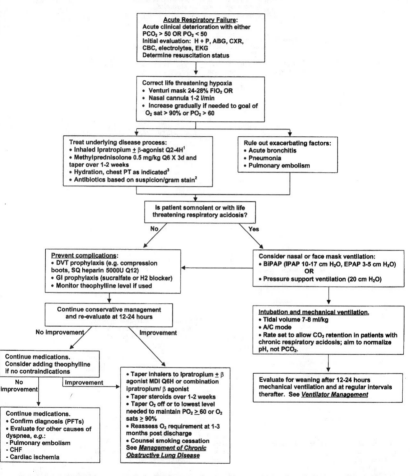

Acute Respiratory Failure:
Acute clinical deterioration with either $PCO_2 > 50$ OR $PO_2 < 50$
Initial evaluation: H + P, ABG, CXR, CBC, electrolytes, EKG
Determine resuscitation status

Correct life threatening hypoxia
- Venturi mask 24-28% FIO_2 OR
- Nasal cannula 1-2 l/min
- Increase gradually if needed to goal of O_2 sat > 90% or $PO_2 > 60$

Treat underlying disease process:
- Inhaled Ipratropium ± β-agonist Q2-4H[1]
- Methylprednisolone 0.5 mg/kg Q6 X 3d and taper over 1-2 weeks
- Hydration, chest PT as indicated[3]
- Antibiotics based on suspicion/gram stain[2]

Rule out exacerbating factors:
- Acute bronchitis
- Pneumonia
- Pulmonary embolism

Is patient somnolent or with life threatening respiratory acidosis?

No / Yes

Prevent complications:
- DVT prophylaxis (e.g. compression boots, SQ heparin 5000U Q12)
- GI prophylaxis (sucralfate or H2 blocker)
- Monitor theophylline level if used

Consider nasal or face mask ventilation:
- BiPAP (IPAP 10-17 cm H_2O, EPAP 3-5 cm H_2O)
   OR
- Pressure support ventilation (20 cm H_2O)

Continue conservative management and re-evaluate at 12-24 hours

No improvement / Improvement

Intubation and mechanical ventilation.
- Tidal volume 7-8 ml/kg
- A/C mode
- Rate set to allow CO_2 retention in patients with chronic respiratory acidosis; aim to normalize pH, not PCO_2.

Continue medications. Consider adding theophylline if no contraindications

No improvement / Improvement

- Taper inhalers to ipratropium ± β agonist MDI Q6H or combination ipratropium/ β agonist
- Taper steroids over 1-2 weeks
- Taper O_2 off or to lowest level needed to maintain $PO_2 \geq 60$ or O_2 sats $\geq$ 90%
- Reassess O_2 requirement at 1-3 months post discharge
- Counsel smoking cessation
See *Management of Chronic Obstructive Lung Disease*

Evaluate for weaning after 12-24 hours mechanical ventilation and at regular intervals therafter. See *Ventilator Management*

Continue medications.
- Confirm diagnosis (PFTs)
- Evaluate for other causes of dyspnea, e.g.:
  - Pulmonary embolism
  - CHF
  - Cardiac ischemia

---

1. Ipratropium bromide MDI 2-6 puffs Q 4-6H or nebulize 0.5 mg solution; Albuterol MDI 2 puffs Q 2-4H or nebulize 0.5 ml of 0.5% solution
2. 7 days of broad spectrum po agent e.g.: doxycline 100 mg bid, trimethoprim sulfasoxazole 1 DS BID, amoxicillin/clavulinic acid 500 mg bid, 2nd generation cephalosporin, clarithromycin 250-500 mg bid, or azithromycin 250 mg, 2 on day 1 followed by 1 qd for 4 days.
3. Chest PT may cause increased hypoxemia.

Curtis JR, Hudson LD. Emergent assessment and management of acute respiratory failure in COPD. Clin Chest Med 15:481-497, 1994
Ferguson GT, Cherniack RM. Management of chronic obstructive pulmonary disease. N Engl J Med 328:1017-1022, 1993

3f: Interstitial Lung Disease (ILD): Diagnostic Evaluation

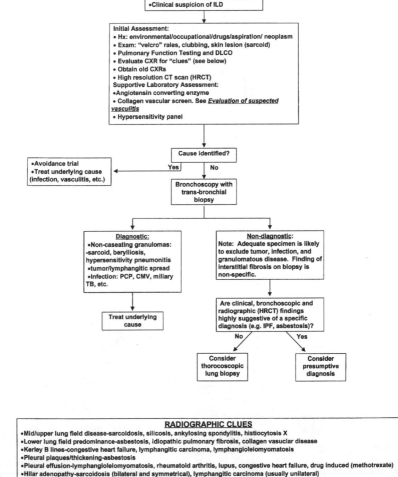

•Symptoms of unexplained dyspnea
•Clinical suspicion of ILD

Initial Assessment:
- Hx: environmental/occupational/drugs/aspiration/ neoplasm
- Exam: "velcro" rales, clubbing, skin lesion (sarcoid)
- Pulmonary Function Testing and DLCO
- Evaluate CXR for "clues" (see below)
- Obtain old CXRs
- High resolution CT scan (HRCT)

Supportive Laboratory Assessment:
- Angiotensin converting enzyme
- Collagen vascular screen. See *Evaluation of suspected vasculitis*
- Hypersensitivity panel

Cause identified?

Yes   No

•Avoidance trial
•Treat underlying cause (infection, vasculitis, etc.)

Bronchoscopy with trans-bronchial biopsy

Diagnostic:
- Non-caseating granulomas:
  - sarcoid, berylliosis, hypersensitivity pneumonitis
- tumor/lymphangitic spread
- Infection: PCP, CMV, miliary TB, etc.

Treat underlying cause

Non-diagnostic:
Note: Adequate specimen is likely to exclude tumor, infection, and granulomatous disease. Finding of interstitial fibrosis on biopsy is non-specific.

Are clinical, bronchoscopic and radiographic (HRCT) findings highly suggestive of a specific diagnosis (e.g. IPF, asbestosis)?

No   Yes

Consider thorocoscopic lung biopsy

Consider presumptive diagnosis

RADIOGRAPHIC CLUES
- Mid/upper lung field disease-sarcoidosis, silicosis, ankylosing spondylitis, histiocytosis X
- Lower lung field predominance-asbestosis, idiopathic pulmonary fibrosis, collagen vasuclar disease
- Kerley B lines-congestive heart failure, lymphangitic carcinoma, lymphangioleiomyomatosis
- Pleural plaques/thickening-asbestosis
- Pleural effusion-lymphangioleiomyomatosis, rheumatoid arthritis, lupus, congestive heart failure, drug induced (methotrexate)
- Hilar adenopathy-sarcoidosis (bilateral and symmetrical), lymphangitic carcinoma (usually unilateral)
- Preserved lung volumes-sarcoidosis, histiocytosis X, lymphangioleiomyomatosis
- Thin-walled cysts (better seen on HRCT)-lymphangioleiomyomatosis, histiocytosis X

Schwarz M. Approach to the understanding, diagnosis and management of interstitial lung disease. In: Interstitial Lung Disease, Schwarz MI and King TE (eds). Mosby Year Book, St Louis, 3rd edition, 1998.

3g: Treatment of Idiopathic Pulmonary Fibrosis

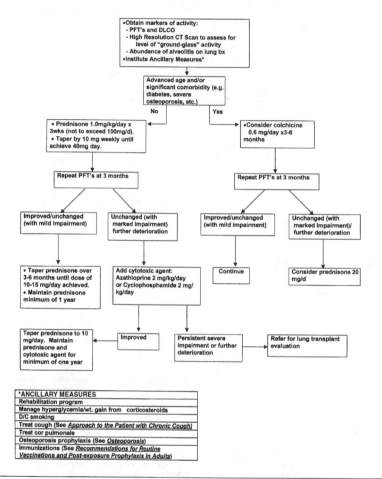

•Obtain markers of activity:
- PFT's and DLCO
- High Resolution CT Scan to assess for level of "ground-glass" activity
- Abundance of alveolitis on lung bx
•Institute Ancillary Measures*

Advanced age and/or significant comorbidity (e.g. diabetes, severe osteoporosis, etc.)

No → • Prednisone 1.0mg/kg/day x 3wks (not to exceed 100mg/d). • Taper by 10 mg weekly until achieve 40mg day.

Yes → •Consider colchicine 0.6 mg/day x3-6 months

Repeat PFT's at 3 months

Repeat PFT's at 3 months

Improved/unchanged (with mild impairment) → • Taper prednisone over 3-6 months until dose of 10-15 mg/day achieved. • Maintain prednisone minimum of 1 year

Unchanged (with marked impairment) further deterioration → Add cytotoxic agent: Azathioprine 2 mg/kg/day or Cyclophosphamide 2 mg/kg/day

Improved/unchanged (with mild impairment) → Continue

Unchanged (with marked impairment)/ further deterioration → Consider prednisone 20 mg/d

Taper prednisone to 10 mg/day. Maintain prednisone and cytotoxic agent for minimum of one year ← Improved

Persistent severe impairment or further deterioration → Refer for lung transplant evaluation

*ANCILLARY MEASURES
Rehabilitation program
Manage hyperglycemia/wt. gain from corticosteroids
D/C smoking
Treat cough (See *Approach to the Patient with Chronic Cough*)
Treat cor pulmonale
Osteoporosis prophylaxis (See *Osteoporosis*)
Immunizations (See *Recommendations for Routine Vaccinations and Post-exposure Prophylaxis in Adults*)

Raghu G. Idiopathic pulmonary fibrosis: a rational clinical approach. Chest 92:148-154, 1987.
Raghu G, Depaso WJ, Cain K, et al. Azathioprine combined with prednisone in the treatment of idiopathic pulmonary fibrosis: a prospective double-blind, randomized, placebo-controlled clinical trial. Am Rev Respir Dis 144: 291-296, 1991.
Reynolds, H.Y. Diagnostic and management strategies for diffuse interstital lung disease. Chest 113:192-202, 1998.

3h: Treatment of Sarcoidosis

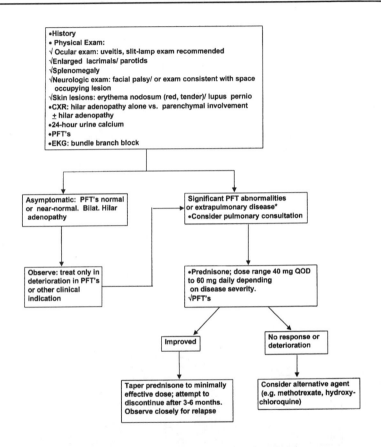

- History
- Physical Exam:
- √ Ocular exam: uveitis, slit-lamp exam recommended
- √Enlarged lacrimals/ parotids
- √Splenomegaly
- √Neurologic exam: facial palsy/ or exam consistent with space occupying lesion
- √Skin lesions: erythema nodosum (red, tender)/ lupus pernio
- CXR: hilar adenopathy alone vs. parenchymal involvement ± hilar adenopathy
- 24-hour urine calcium
- PFT's
- EKG: bundle branch block

Asymptomatic: PFT's normal or near-normal. Bilat. Hilar adenopathy

Significant PFT abnormalities or extrapulmonary disease*
- Consider pulmonary consultation

Observe: treat only in deterioration in PFT's or other clinical indication

- Prednisone; dose range 40 mg QOD to 60 mg daily depending on disease severity.
√PFT's

Improved

No response or deterioration

Taper prednisone to minimally effective dose; attempt to discontinue after 3-6 months. Observe closely for relapse

Consider alternative agent (e.g. methotrexate, hydroxychloroquine)

*Extrapulmonary Disease in Sarcoidosis:
Includes central nervous system involvement, cardiac disease, liver involvement with marked derangements in liver function studies, posterior chamber uveitis, severe and disfiguring skin lesions, hypercalcemia refractory to dietary manipulation, or profound constitutional symptoms (weight loss, fevers, nightsweats, severe fatigue). Topical corticosteroids may be used for milder forms of cutaneous sarcoid and for anterior chamber uveitis. Nonsteroidal antiinflammatory agents may be used for painful erythema nodosum.

Kotloff RM and Rossman MD. Sarcoidosis. Immunol Allerg Clin North Amer 12:421-449, 1992.

3i: Pulmonary Hypertension

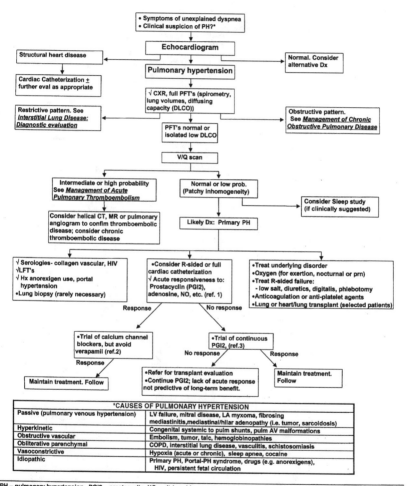

- Symptoms of unexplained dyspnea
- Clinical suspicion of PH?*

Echocardiogram

Structural heart disease

Normal. Consider alternative Dx

Pulmonary hypertension

Cardiac Catheterization ± further eval as appropriate

√ CXR, full PFT's (spirometry, lung volumes, diffusing capacity (DLCO))

Restrictive pattern. See *Interstitial Lung Disease: Diagnostic evaluation*

Obstructive pattern. See *Management of Chronic Obstructive Pulmonary Disease*

PFT's normal or isolated low DLCO

V/Q scan

Intermediate or high probability See *Management of Acute Pulmonary Thromboembolism*

Normal or low prob. (Patchy inhomogeneity)

Consider Sleep study (if clinically suggested)

Consider helical CT, MR or pulmonary angiogram to confirm thromboembolic disease; consider chronic thromboembolic disease

Likely Dx: Primary PH

- √ Serologies- collagen vascular, HIV
- √ LFT's
- √ Hx anorexigen use, portal hypertension
- Lung biopsy (rarely necessary)

- Consider R-sided or full cardiac catheterization
- √ Acute responsiveness to: Prostacyclin (PGI2), adenosine, NO, etc. (ref. 1)

- Treat underlying disorder
- Oxygen (for exertion, nocturnal or prn)
- Treat R-sided failure:
  - low salt, diuretics, digitalis, phlebotomy
- Anticoagulation or anti-platelet agents
- Lung or heart/lung transplant (selected patients)

Response   No response

- Trial of calcium channel blockers, but avoid verapamil (ref.2)

- Trial of continuous PGI2, (ref.3)

No response   Response

Response

Maintain treatment. Follow

- Refer for transplant evaluation
- Continue PGI2; lack of acute response not predictive of long-term benefit.

Maintain treatment. Follow

*CAUSES OF PULMONARY HYPERTENSION	
Passive (pulmonary venous hypertension)	LV failure, mitral disease, LA myxoma, fibrosing mediastinitis, mediastinal/hilar adenopathy (i.e. tumor, sarcoidosis)
Hyperkinetic	Congenital systemic to pulm shunts, pulm AV malformations
Obstructive vascular	Embolism, tumor, talc, hemoglobinopathies
Obliterative parenchymal	COPD, interstitial lung disease, vasculitis, schistosomiasis
Vasoconstrictive	Hypoxia (acute or chronic), sleep apnea, cocaine
Idiopathic	Primary PH, Portal-PH syndrome, drugs (e.g. anorexigens), HIV, persistent fetal circulation

PH – pulmonary hypertension. PGI2 – prostacyclin, NO – nitric oxide
1. Palevsky HI. The treatment of Pulmonary Hypertension. *In:* Pulmonary Pharmacology and Therapeutics, AR Leff (ed), New York, McGraw Hill, 1996, pp. 1099-1109.
2. Rich S, Kaufmann E, Levy PA. The effect of high doses of calcium-channel blockers on survival in primary pulmonary hypertension. N Engl J Med 327:76-81, 1992.
3. Barst RJ, et al. A comparison of continuous intravenous epoprostenol (prostacyclin) with conventional therapy for primary pulmonary hypertension. N Engl J Med 334:296-301, 1996.

3j: Pleural Effusion

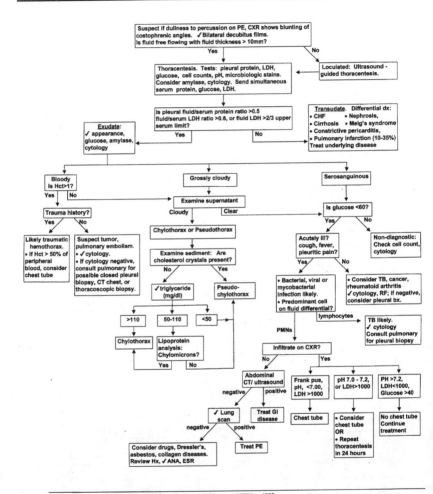

Suspect if dullness to percussion on PE, CXR shows blunting of costophrenic angles. ✓ Bilateral decubitus films.
Is fluid free flowing with fluid thickness > 10mm?

Yes → Thoracentesis. Tests: pleural protein, LDH, glucose, cell counts, pH, microbiologic stains. Consider amylase, cytology. Send simultaneous serum protein, glucose, LDH.

No → Loculated: Ultrasound - guided thoracentesis.

Is pleural fluid/serum protein ratio >0.5 fluid/serum LDH ratio >0.6, or fluid LDH >2/3 upper serum limit?

Transudate. Differential dx:
- CHF
- Nephrosis,
- Cirrhosis
- Meig's syndrome
- Constrictive pericarditis,
- Pulmonary infarction (10-35%)
Treat underlying disease

Yes → Exudate: ✓ appearance, glucose, amylase, cytology

Bloody Is Hct>1?
Yes / No

Trauma history?
Yes / No

Likely traumatic hemothorax.
- If Hct > 50% of peripheral blood, consider chest tube

Suspect tumor, pulmonary embolism.
- ✓ cytology.
- If cytology negative, consult pulmonary for possible closed pleural biopsy, CT chest, or thoracoscopic biopsy.

Grossly cloudy

Examine supernatant
Cloudy / Clear

Chylothorax or Pseudothorax

Examine sediment: Are cholesterol crystals present?
No / Yes

✓ triglyceride (mg/dl) / Pseudo-chylothorax

>110 / 50-110 / <50

Chylothorax / Lipoprotein analysis: Chylomicrons?
Yes / No

Serosanguineous

Is glucose <60?
Yes / No

Acutely ill? cough, fever, pleuritic pain?
Yes / No

Non-diagnostic: Check cell count, cytology

- Bacterial, viral or mycobacterial infection likely.
- Predominant cell on fluid differential?

- Consider TB, cancer, rheumatoid arthritis ✓ cytology, RF; if negative, consider pleural bx.

lymphocytes → TB likely. ✓ cytology Consult pulmonary for pleural biopsy

PMNs

Infiltrate on CXR?
No / Yes

Abdominal CT/ ultrasound
negative / positive

✓ Lung scan / Treat GI disease
negative / positive

Consider drugs, Dressler's, asbestos, collagen diseases. Review Hx, ✓ ANA, ESR

Treat PE

Frank pus, pH, <7.00, LDH >1000 → Chest tube

pH 7.0 - 7.2, or LDH>1000 → • Consider chest tube OR • Repeat thoracentesis in 24 hours

PH >7.2, LDH<1000, Glucose >40 → No chest tube Continue treatment

1. Light, RW. Pleural Diseases 3rd edition. Baltimore, Williams and Wilkins, 1995.
2. Guidelines for Thoracentesis and Needle Biopsy of the Pleura. Am Rev Respir Dis. 140:257-258. 1989.

3k: Approach to the Patient with Chronic Cough

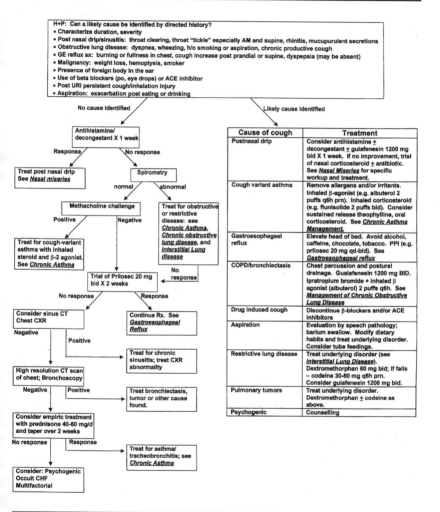

H+P: Can a likely cause be identified by directed history?
- Characterize duration, severity
- Post nasal drip/sinusitis: throat clearing, throat "tickle" especially AM and supine, rhinitis, mucupurulent secretions
- Obstructive lung disease: dyspnea, wheezing, h/o smoking or aspiration, chronic productive cough
- GE reflux sx: burning or fullness in chest, cough increase post prandial or supine, dyspepsia (may be absent)
- Malignancy: weight loss, hemoptysis, smoker
- Presence of foreign body in the ear
- Use of beta blockers (po, eye drops) or ACE inhibitor
- Post URI persistent cough/inhalation injury
- Aspiration: exacerbation post eating or drinking

No cause identified

Antihistamine/decongestant X 1 week

Response → Treat post nasal drip See *Nasal miseries*

No response → Spirometry

normal → Methacholine challenge

Positive → Treat for cough-variant asthma with inhaled steroid and β-2 agonist. See *Chronic Asthma*

Negative → Trial of Prilosec 20 mg bid X 2 weeks

abnormal → Treat for obstructive or restrictive disease: see *Chronic Asthma, Chronic obstructive lung disease,* and *Interstitial Lung disease*

No response → Trial of Prilosec 20 mg bid X 2 weeks

No response → Consider sinus CT Chest CXR

Response → Continue Rx. See *Gastroesophageal Reflux*

Negative → High resolution CT scan of chest; Bronchoscopy

Positive → Treat for chronic sinusitis; treat CXR abnormality

Negative → Consider empiric treatment with prednisone 40-60 mg/d and taper over 2 weeks

Positive → Treat bronchiectasis, tumor or other cause found.

No response → Consider: Psychogenic Occult CHF Multifactorial

Response → Treat for asthma/tracheobronchitis; see *Chronic Asthma*

Likely cause identified

Cause of cough	Treatment
Postnasal drip	Consider antihistamine ± decongestant ± guaifenesin 1200 mg bid X 1 week. If no improvement, trial of nasal corticosteroid ± antibiotic. See *Nasal Miseries* for specific workup and treatment.
Cough variant asthma	Remove allergens and/or irritants. Inhaled β-agonist (e.g. albuterol 2 puffs q6h prn). Inhaled corticosteroid (e.g. flunisolide 2 puffs bid). Consider sustained release theophylline, oral corticosteroid. See *Chronic Asthma Management.*
Gastroesophageal reflux	Elevate head of bed. Avoid alcohol, caffeine, chocolate, tobacco. PPI (e.g. prilosec 20 mg qd-bid). See *Gastroesophageal reflux*
COPD/bronchiectasis	Chest percussion and postural drainage. Guaifenesin 1200 mg BID. Ipratropium bromide + inhaled β agonist (albuterol) 2 puffs q6h. See *Management of Chronic Obstructive Lung Disease*
Drug induced cough	Discontinue β-blockers and/or ACE inhibitors
Aspiration	Evaluation by speech pathology; barium swallow. Modify dietary habits and treat underlying disorder. Consider tube feedings.
Restrictive lung disease	Treat underlying disorder (see *Interstitial Lung Disease*). Dextromethorphan 60 mg bid; if fails – codeine 30-60 mg q6h prn. Consider guaifenesin 1200 mg bid.
Pulmonary tumors	Treat underlying disorder. Dextromethorphan ± codeine as above.
Psychogenic	Counselling

Patrick H, Patrick F. Chronic cough. Med Clin North Amer 79:361-372, 1995.
Pratter MR, Bartter T, Akers S, et al. An algorithmic approach to chronic cough. Ann Intern Med 119:977-983, 1993.
Irwin RS, Curley FJ. The treatment of cough, a comprehensive review. Chest 99:1477-1484, 1991.

3I: Solitary Pulmonary Nodule

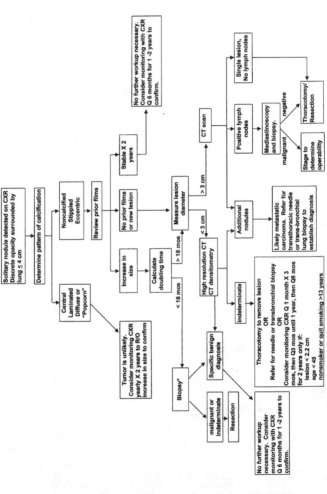

*Controversial. Some authors suggest fiberoptic bronchoscopy (for central lesions 2-4 cm) or transthoracic needle biopsy (for peripheral lesions or if bronchoscopy is negative). Others suggest proceeding directly to resection, especially if clinical suspicion for malignancy is high. Isolated lesions with rapid doubling times (< 7-21 days) are less likely to be malignant.

Midthun DE. Solitary Pulmonary nodule. www.chestnet.org/lesson18.html, 1997
Midthun DE, Swensen SJ, Jett FR. Approach to the Solitary Pulmonary Nodule. Mayo Clin Proc 68:378-385, 1993
Lillington GA. Management of Solitary Pulmonary Nodules. Dis Mon 37: 278-310, 1991
Viggiano RW, Swensen SJ, Rosenow EC. Evaluation and Management of Solitary and Multiple Pulmonary Nodules. Clin Chest Med 13:83-92, 1992

3m: Workup and Treatment of Persistent and Intractable Hiccups

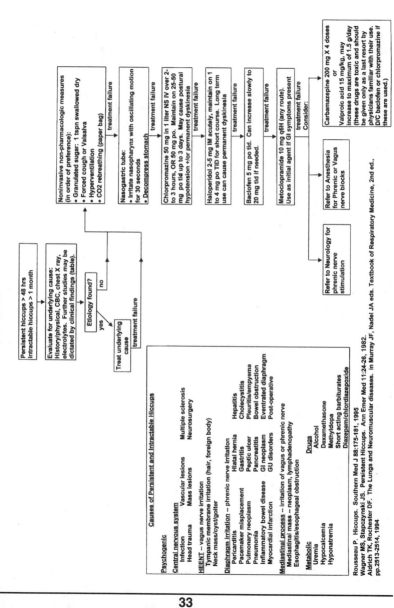

Persistent hiccups > 48 hrs
Intractable hiccups > 1 month

Evaluate for underlying cause: History/physical, CBC, chest X ray, electrolytes. Further studies may be dictated by clinical findings (table).

Etiology found?

yes → Treat underlying cause → treatment failure

no →

Noninvasive non-pharmacologic measures (in order of preference):
• Granulated sugar: 1 tspn swallowed dry
• Forced cough or Valsalva
• Hyperventilation
• CO2 rebreathing (paper bag)

treatment failure

Nasogastric tube:
• Irritate nasopharynx with oscillating motion for 30 seconds
• Decompress stomach

treatment failure

Chlorpromazine 50 mg in 1 liter NS IV over 2- to 3 hours, OR 50 mg po. Maintain on 25-50 mg po tid up to 3 days. May cause postural hypotension +/or permanent dyskinesia

treatment failure

Haloperidol 2-5 mg IM acutely, maintain on 1 to 4 mg po TID for short course. Long term use can cause permanent dyskinesia

treatment failure

Baclofen 5 mg po tid. Can increase slowly to 20 mg tid if needed.

treatment failure

Metoclopramide 10 mg q6H (any route). Use as initial agent if GI symptoms present

treatment failure
Consider:

Refer to Anesthesia for Phrenic or Vagus nerve blocks

Refer to Neurology for phrenic nerve stimulation

Carbamazepine 200 mg X 4 doses
or
Valproic acid 15 mg/Kg, may increase to maximum of 1.5 g/day (these drugs are toxic and should be given only as a last resort by physicians familiar with their use. D/C baclofen or chlorpromazine if these are used.)

Causes of Persistent and Intractable Hiccups

Psychogenic

Central nervous system
Infection   Vascular lesions   Multiple sclerosis
Head trauma   Mass lesions   Neurosurgery

HEENT -- vagus nerve irritation
Tympanic membrane irritation (hair, foreign body)
Neck mass/cyst/goiter

Diaphragm Irritation -- phrenic nerve irritation
Pericarditis   Hiatal hernia   Hepatitis
Pacemaker misplacement Gastritis   Cholecystitis
Pulmonary neoplasm   Peptic ulcer   Pleuritis/empyema
Pneumonia   Pancreatitis   Bowel obstruction
Inflammatory bowel disease GI disorders   Eventrated diaphragm
Myocardial infarction GU disorders   Post-operative

Mediastinal process -- irritation of vagus or phrenic nerve
Mediastinal mass -- neoplasm, lymphadenopathy
Esophagitis/esophageal obstruction

Metabolic   Drugs
Uremia   Alcohol
Hypocalcemia   Dexamethasone
Hyponatremia   Methyldopa
                      Short acting barbiturates
                      Diazepam/chlordiazepoxide

Rousseau P. Hiccups. Southern Med J 88:175-181, 1995
Wagner MS, Stapczynski JS. Persistent Hiccups. Ann Emer Med 11:24-26, 1982.
Aldrich TK, Rochester DF. The Lungs and Neuromuscular diseases. In Murray JF, Nadel JA eds. Textbook of Respiratory Medicine, 2nd ed., pp.2513-2514, 1994

3n: Evaluation and Management of Hemoptysis

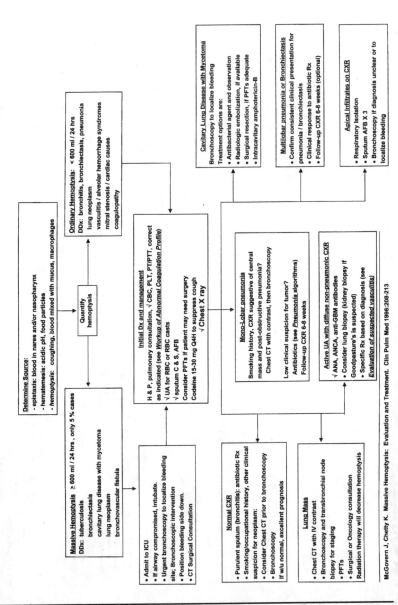

Determine Source:
- epistaxis: blood in nares and/or nasopharynx
- hematemesis: acidic pH, food particles
- *hemoptysis*: coughing, blood mixed with mucus, macrophages

Quantify hemoptysis

Massive Hemoptysis: ≥ 600 ml / 24 hrs, only 5 % cases
DDx: tuberculosis
bronchiectasis
cavitary lung disease with mycetoma
lung neoplasm
bronchovascular fistula

- Admit to ICU
- If airway compromised, intubate.
- Urgent bronchoscopy to localize bleeding site; Bronchoscopic intervention
- Position bleeding side down.
- CT Surgical Consultation

Ordinary Hemoptysis: < 600 ml / 24 hrs
DDx: bronchitis, bronchiectasis, pneumonia
lung neoplasm
vasculitis / alveolar hemorrhage syndromes
mitral stenosis / cardiac causes
coagulopathy

Initial Dx and management
H & P, pulmonary consultation, √ CBC, PLT, PT/PTT, correct as indicated (see *Workup of Abnormal Coagulation Profile*)
√ UA for RBC or RBC casts
√ sputum C & S, AFB
Consider PFTs if patient may need surgery
Codeine 15-30 mg Q4H to suppress cough
√ Chest X ray

Normal CXR
- Purulent sputum (bronchitis): antibiotic Rx
- Smoking/occupational history, other clinical suspicion for neoplasm:
- Consider Chest CT prior to bronchoscopy
- Bronchoscopy
If w/u normal, excellent prognosis

Lung Mass
- Chest CT with IV contrast
- Bronchoscopy and transbronchial node biopsy for staging
- PFTs
- Surgical or Oncology consultation
Radiation therapy will decrease hemoptysis

Mono-Lobar pneumonia
Smoking history, CXR suggestive of central mass and post-obstructive pneumonia?
Chest CT with contrast, then bronchoscopy

Low clinical suspicion for tumor?
Antibiotics (see *Pneumonia* algorithms)
Follow-up CXR 6-8 weeks

Active UA with diffuse non-pneumonic CXR
√ ANA, ANCA, anti-GBM antibodies
- Consider lung biopsy (kidney biopsy if Goodpasture's is suspected)
- Specific Rx based on diagnosis (see *Evaluation of suspected vasculitis*)

Cavitary Lung Disease with Mycetoma
Bronchoscopy to localize bleeding
Treatment options are:
- Antibacterial agent and observation
- Radiologic embolization, if available
- Surgical resection, if PFTs adequate
- Intracavitary amphotericin-B

Multilobar pneumonia or Bronchiectasis
- Confirm consistent clinical presentation for pneumonia / bronchiectasis
- Clinical response to antibiotic Rx
- Follow-up CXR 6-8 weeks (optional)

Apical Infiltrates on CXR
- Respiratory Isolation
- Sputum AFB X 3
- Bronchoscopy if diagnosis unclear or to localize bleeding

McGovern J, Chetty K. Massive Hemoptysis: Evaluation and Treatment. Clin Pulm Med 1996:208-213

3o: Management of Community Acquired Pneumonia

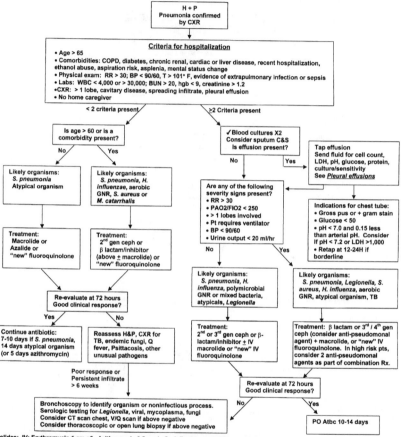

H + P
Pneumonia confirmed
by CXR

Criteria for hospitalization

- Age > 65
- Comorbidities: COPD, diabetes, chronic renal, cardiac or liver disease, recent hospitalization, ethanol abuse, aspiration risk, asplenia, mental status change
- Physical exam: RR > 30; BP < 90/60, T > 101° F, evidence of extrapulmonary infection or sepsis
- Labs: WBC < 4,000 or > 30,000; BUN > 20, hgb < 9, creatinine > 1.2
- CXR: > 1 lobe, cavitary disease, spreading infiltrate, pleural effusion
- No home caregiver

< 2 criteria present → Is age > 60 or is a comorbidity present?

≥2 Criteria present → ✓ Blood cultures X2 / Consider sputum C&S / Is effusion present?

No:
Likely organisms:
S. pneumonia
Atypical organism

Treatment:
Macrolide or
Azalide or
"new" fluoroquinolone

Yes:
Likely organisms:
S. pneumonia, H. influenzae, aerobic GNR, S. aureus or M. catarrhalis

Treatment:
2nd gen ceph or
β lactam/inhibitor
(above ± macrolide) or
"new" fluoroquinolone

Re-evaluate at 72 hours
Good clinical response?

Yes:
Continue antibiotic:
7-10 days if S. pneumonia,
14 days atypical organism
(or 5 days azithromycin)

No:
Reassess H&P, CXR for TB, endemic fungi, Q fever, Psittacosis, other unusual pathogens

Poor response or
Persistent infiltrate
> 6 weeks

Bronchoscopy to identify organism or noninfectious process.
Serologic testing for Legionella, viral, mycoplasma, fungi
Consider CT scan chest, V/Q scan if above negative
Consider thoracoscopic or open lung biopsy if above negative

(effusion present) **Yes:**
Tap effusion
Send fluid for cell count, LDH, pH, glucose, protein, culture/sensitivity
See *Pleural effusions*

No:
Are any of the following severity signs present?
- RR > 30
- PAO2/FIO2 < 250
- > 1 lobes involved
- Pt requires ventilator
- BP < 90/60
- Urine output < 20 ml/hr

Indications for chest tube:
- Gross pus or + gram stain
- Glucose < 50
- pH < 7.0 and 0.15 less than arterial pH. Consider if pH < 7.2 or LDH >1,000
- Retap at 12-24H if borderline

No:
Likely organisms:
S. pneumonia, H. influenza, polymicrobial GNR or mixed bacteria, atypicals, Legionella

Treatment:
2nd or 3rd gen ceph or β-lactam/inhibitor ± IV macrolide or "new" IV fluoroquinolone

Yes:
Likely organisms:
S. pneumonia, Legionella, S. aureus, H. influenza, aerobic GNR, atypical organism, TB

Treatment: β lactam or 3rd / 4th gen ceph (consider anti-pseudomonal agent) + macrolide, or "new" IV fluoroquinolone. In high risk pts, consider 2 anti-pseudomonal agents as part of combination Rx.

Re-evaluate at 72 hours
Good clinical response?

No / **Yes** → PO Atbc 10-14 days

Macrolides: IV: Erythromycin 1 gm q6. Azithromycin 0.5 g qd. Oral: Erythromycin 500 mg qid, Clarithromycin 500 mg bid, Azithromycin 0.5 g po day 1, then 250 mg qd X 4 days

β lactam/inhibitor: Amoxicillin/clavulanate 875 mg bid, Ampicillin/sulbactam 1.5–3.0 g q6h, (see antipseudomonals for ticar/clav and pip/tazo)
IV 2nd gen cephalosporin: Cefuroxime 750 mg q8h; Cefotetan 2 g q12h; Cefoxitin 2g q8h. Oral: Cefuroxime or Cefaclor 250-500 mg bid
IV 3rd gen cephalosporin: Cefotaxime 2 g q4-8h; Ceftriaxone 1-2 g qd
Antipseudomonals: Ceftazadime 2g q8, Piperacillin/tazobactam 4.5g q6h, Ticarcillin/clavulanate 3.1g q4-6h, Imipenem 0.5gQ6h, Ciprofloxacin 400mg IV q12h or 750mg po Q12h, Trovafloxacin 300 mg qd, Levofloxacin 500 mg qd, Cefepime1.0-2.0 g q12h
Aminoglycosides: adjust to level and renal function. Gentamicin or Tobramycin 3-5 mg/kg/d as single daily dose or divided into 2 or 3 doses. Amikacin 7.5mg/kg q12, not to exceed 1.5g/day.
"new" fluoroquinolones: Grepafloxacin 600 mg po qd, Levofloxacin 500 mg qd (IV or po), Sparfloxacin 400 mg load, then 200 mg po qd, Trovafloxacin 200 mg po qd or 200 – 300 mg IV qd
*Some experts combine antipseudomonal β lactams with quinalone as an alternative to aminoglycosides in patients with renal impairment.
ATS Statement. Guidelines for the initial management of adults with community acquired pneumonia: Diagnosis, assessment of severity, and initial antimicrobial therapy. Am Rev Resp Dis 148: 1418, 1993

3p: Nosocomial Pneumonia

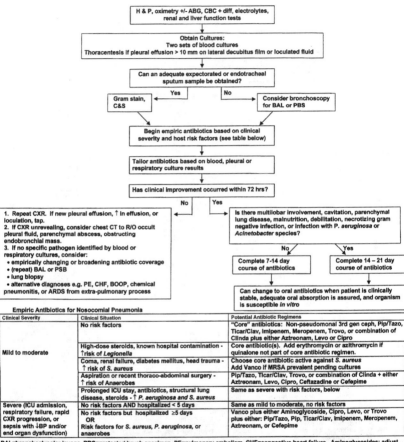

H & P, oximetry +/- ABG, CBC + diff, electrolytes, renal and liver function tests

↓

Obtain Cultures:
Two sets of blood cultures
Thoracentesis if pleural effusion > 10 mm on lateral decubitus film or loculated fluid

↓

Can an adequate expectorated or endotracheal sputum sample be obtained?

Yes → Gram stain, C&S

No → Consider bronchoscopy for BAL or PBS

↓

Begin empiric antibiotics based on clinical severity and host risk factors (see table below)

↓

Tailor antibiotics based on blood, pleural or respiratory culture results

↓

Has clinical improvement occurred within 72 hrs?

No:
1. Repeat CXR. If new pleural effusion, ↑ in effusion, or loculation, tap.
2. If CXR unrevealing, consider chest CT to R/O occult pleural fluid, parenchymal abscess, obstructing endobronchial mass.
3. If no specific pathogen identified by blood or respiratory cultures, consider:
 • empirically changing or broadening antibiotic coverage
 • (repeat) BAL or PSB
 • lung biopsy
 • alternative diagnoses e.g. PE, CHF, BOOP, chemical pneumonitis, or ARDS from extra-pulmonary process

Yes: Is there multilobar involvement, cavitation, parenchymal lung disease, malnutrition, debilitation, necrotizing gram negative infection, or infection with P. aeruginosa or Acinetobacter species?

No → Complete 7-14 day course of antibiotics

Yes → Complete 14 – 21 day course of antibiotics

↓

Can change to oral antibiotics when patient is clinically stable, adequate oral absorption is assured, and organism is susceptible in vitro

Empiric Antibiotics for Nosocomial Pneumonia

Clinical Severity	Clinical Situation	Potential Antibiotic Regimens
Mild to moderate	No risk factors	"Core" antibiotics: Non-pseudomonal 3rd gen ceph, Pip/Tazo, Ticar/Clav, Imipenem, Meropenem, Trovo, or combination of Clinda plus either Aztreonam, Levo or Cipro
	High-dose steroids, known hospital contamination - ↑risk of Legionella	Core antibiotic(s). Add erythromycin or azithromycin if quinalone not part of core antibiotic regimen.
	Coma, renal failure, diabetes mellitus, head trauma - ↑ risk of S. aureus	Choose core antibiotic active against S. aureus Add Vanco if MRSA prevalent pending cultures
	Aspiration or recent thoraco-abdominal surgery - ↑ risk of Anaerobes	Pip/Tazo, Ticar/Clav, Trovo, or combination of Clinda + either Aztreonam, Levo, Cipro, Ceftazadine or Cefepime
	Prolonged ICU stay, antibiotics, structural lung disease, steroids - ↑ P. aeruginosa and S. aureus	Same as severe with risk factors, below
Severe (ICU admission, respiratory failure, rapid CXR progression, or sepsis with ↓BP and/or end organ dysfunction)	No risk factors AND hospitalized < 5 days	Same as mild to moderate, no risk factors
	No risk factors but hospitalized ≥5 days OR Risk factors for S. aureus, P. aeruginosa, or anaerobes	Vanco plus either Aminoglycoside, Cipro, Levo, or Trovo plus either: Pip/Tazo, Pip, Ticar/Clav, Imipenem, Meropenem, Aztreonam, or Cefepime

BAL=bronchoalveolar lavage, PBS=protected brush specimen, PE=pulmonary embolism, CHF=congestive heart failure. Aminoglycosides: adjust to level and renal function. Gentamicin or Tobramycin 3-5 mg/kg/d as single daily dose or divided into 2 or 3 doses. Amikacin 7.5mg/kg q12, not to exceed 1.5 g/day. Aztreonam 1g q8h-2g q6h, Azithromycin 500 mg qd, Cefepime 1.0-2.0 g q12h, Clinda=clindamycin 600 mg q8h, Cipro=ciprofloxacin 400-750 mg q12h, Trovo=trovafloxacin 300 mg qd, Levo=levofloxacin 500 mg qd, Erythromycin 1.0g q6h, Nonpseudomonal 3rd gen Ceph=ceftriaxone 1-2 g qd, cefotaxime 2 g Q4-8, Pip/Tazo=piperacillin/tazobactam 3.375g q6h (antipseudomonal dose-4.5g q6h), Ticar/Clav=ticarcillin/clavulanate 3.1g q4-6h, Vanco=vancomycin 1.0g q12h, Pip=piperacillin 4g q6h, Imipenem 0.5 g q6h, Meropenem 0.5-1.0 g q8h

Hospital-acquired Pneumonia in Adults: Diagnosis, Assessment of Severity, Initial Antimicrobial Therapy, and Preventative Strategies. A Consensus Statement. Am J Respir Crit Care Med 153: 1711, 1996

3q: Pneumonia in the Immunocompromised Host

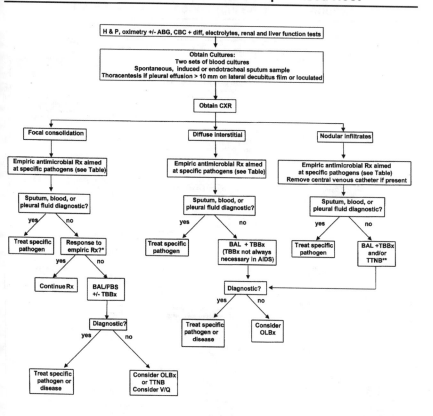

* If patient acutely ill and/or has a rapidly progressive process, may need to proceed directly to diagnostic procedure.
** TTNB especially useful if lesions are peripheral.

Abbreviations: BAL=bronchoalveolar lavage, PBS=protected brush specimen, TBBx =transbronchial biopsy, TTNB=transthoracic thin needle biopsy, V/Q=ventilation/perfusion scan, OLBx=open lung or thoracoscopic biopsy

Shelhamer, JH, moderator. NIH Conference: Respiratory disease in the immunocompromised patient. Ann Intern Med 117: 415, 1992

3r: Differential Diagnosis and Empiric Therapy for Pneumonia in the Immunocompromised Host

CXR Abnormality	Non-infectious Etiologies	Infectious Etiologies	Empiric Therapy
Focal Consolidation	Pulmonary embolism Pulmonary hemorrhage Tumor Less likely: 　Drug-induced 　Radiation-induced	**Bacterial** • Consider *S. pneumoniae, H. influenzae, Legionella pneumophila,* and *Mycoplasma pneumoniae* if acquired in community • Consider *S. aureus* and GNRs if acquired nosocomially Typical and atypical mycobacteria **Fungal:** *Aspergillus* species, *Histoplasma capsulatum, Cryptococcus neoformans, Coccidiodes immitis* *Nocardia asteroides* Less likely: *Pneumocystis carinii,* viral	**Community acquired:** • Macrolide ± 2nd gen ceph, non-pseudomonal 3rd gen ceph, Amp/Sulb, or "new" quinalone **Nosocomial:** • Non-pseudomonal 3rd gen ceph, Pip/Tazo, Ticar/Clav, Imipenem, Meropenem, Trovo, or combination of Clinda plus either Aztreonam, Levo, Cipro, Ceftazadine or Cefepime • Add Vanco if high incidence of MRSA • Add AG if severely ill • Add Ampho B if acutely ill and prolonged immunosupression and broad spectrum antibiotic use
Nodular Infiltrates	Tumor BOOP	Fungal: Aspergillus species, *Histoplasma capsulatum, Cryptococcus neoformans, Coccidiodes immitis* *Nocardia asteroides* Bacterial (especially septic emboli secondary to a central intravenous catheter) Typical and atypical mycobacteria Less likely: *Pneumocystis carinii, Legionella micdadei, Rhodococcus equi*	Ampho B Add Vanco + Gent if central venous catheter in place Consider TMP/S if severely ill while awaiting diagnostic evaluation
Diffuse Infiltrates	• Pulmonary edema • Drug-induced • Leukoagglutination reaction (Consider when syndrome occurs acutely following transfusion) • Radiation-induced • Tumor • Kaposis sarcoma (Consider in AIDS patient with skin or mucous membrane lesions) • Pulmonary hemorrhage • BOOP	• *Pneumocystis carinii* • Viral 　-Consider influenza if community acquired and appropriate season 　-Consider CMV in transplant population. CMV only rarely a true pulmonary pathogen in AIDS 　-Less common: VZV, HSV • Fungal: *Histoplasma capsulatum, Cryptococcus neoformans* • *Toxoplasma gondii* • Typical and atypical mycobacteria MTb commonly presents with diffuse infiltrates in advanced immunodeficiency • Bacterial: *Legionella pneumphila, Mycoplasma pneumoniae, Chlamydia pneumonia*	TMP/S ± Macrolide Add Ganciclovir in transplant patients if appropriate risk factors are present

<u>Abbreviations</u>: GNR=gram negative rod, CMV=cytomegalovirus, VZV=varicella zoster virus, HSV=herpes simplex virus, MTb=*Mycobacterium tuberculosis*, BOOP=bronchiolitis obliterans with organizing pneumonia, Ceph=cephalosporin, Amp/Sulb=ampicillin/sulbactam, Pip/Tazo=piperacillin/tazobactam, Ticar/Clav=ticarcillin/clavulanate, Clinda=clindamycin, Vanco=vancomycin, Pip=piperacillin, AG=aminoglycoside, Gent=gentamicin, TMP/S=trimethoprim sulfamethoxazole, Ampho B=amphotericin B
<u>Reference</u>: Shelhamer, JH, moderator. NIH Conference: Respiratory disease in the immunocompromised patient. Ann Intern Med 117: 415, 1992

3s: Tuberculosis Treatment

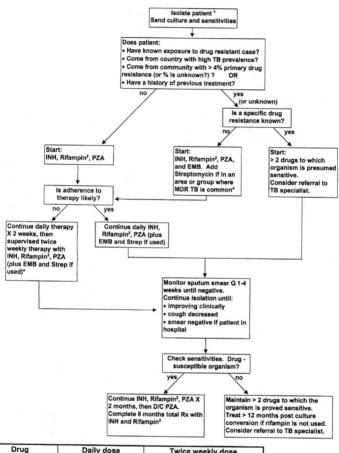

Isolate patient [1]
Send culture and sensitivities

Does patient:
- Have known exposure to drug resistant case?
- Come from country with high TB prevalence?
- Come from community with > 4% primary drug resistance (or % is unknown?) ?   OR
- Have a history of previous treatment?

no → / yes (or unknown)

Is a specific drug resistance known?
no / yes

Start:
INH, Rifampin[2], PZA

Start:
INH, Rifampin[2], PZA, and EMB. Add Streptomycin if in an area or group where MDR TB is common*

Start:
> 2 drugs to which organism is presumed sensitive. Consider referral to TB specialist.

Is adherence to therapy likely?
no / yes

Continue daily therapy X 2 weeks, then supervised twice weekly therapy with INH, Rifampin[2], PZA (plus EMB and Strep if used)*

Continue daily INH, Rifampin[2], PZA (plus EMB and Strep if used)

Monitor sputum smear Q 1-4 weeks until negative.
Continue isolation until:
- improving clinically
- cough decreased
- smear negative if patient in hospital

Check sensitivities. Drug - susceptible organism?
yes / no

Continue INH, Rifampin[2], PZA X 2 months, then D/C PZA. Complete 6 months total Rx with INH and Rifampin[2]

Maintain > 2 drugs to which the organism is proved sensitive. Treat > 12 months post culture conversion if rifampin is not used. Consider referral to TB specialist.

Drug	Daily dose	Twice weekly dose
INH (isoniazid)	300 mg	15 mg/kg (per dose), max 900 mg
Rifampin	600 mg (450 mg if < 50 kg)	600 mg (per dose)
PZA (pyrizinamide)	25 - 30 mg/kg	50 mg/kg (per dose), max 3 gm
EMB (ethambutol)	15 mg/kg	50 mg/kg (per dose)
Strep (streptomycin)	0.7-1.0 g	0.7-1.0 g (per dose)

1. Isolate in private room with negative airflow or recirculated through HEPA filter ± UV light source
2. Rifabutin 300 mg qd should be substituted for rifampin in HIV positive patients receiving protease inhibitors or non-nucleoside reverse transcriptase inhibitors (NNRTis). See *Antiretroviral Agents* for listing of these agents.
ATS/Centers for Disease Control. Treatment of tuberculosis and tuberculosis infection in adults and children. Am Rev Respir Dis 149: 1359-1374; 1994
Center for Disease Control. Initial therapy for tuberculosis in the era of multidrug resistance. MMWR 421 (no. RR-7):1-8, 1993

3t: Tuberculosis Prophylaxis

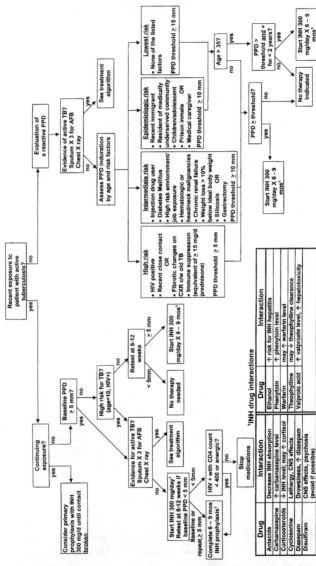

1. 9 to 12 mos if HIV+. Some experts recommend a regimen of daily rifampin 600 mg and PZA 20 mg/kg for 2 months. Rifabutin 300 mg qd should be substituted for rifampin in HIV positive patients receiving protease inhibitors or non-nucleoside reverse transcriptase inhibitors (NNRTIs). Monitor for adherence and side effects q 30d. Consider monthly LFT if age >35 +/or liver dx. INH interaction with other drugs[1], or "regular" ETOH use. Recommendations are currently being updated, check www.PocketDoctor.com for changes. INH - Isoniazid. Pyridoxine (vitamin B6) 25–50 mg qd should be given concommitantly to patients prone to neuropathy (ETOH abuse, diabetes mellitus).

American Thoracic Society/Centers for Disease Control. Diagnostic standards and classification of tuberculosis. Am Rev Respir Dis 142:725-735, 1990
American Thoracic Society/Centers for Disease Control. Treatment of tuberculosis and tuberculosis infection in adults and children. Am Rev Respir Dis 149: 1359-1374; 1994
Centers for Disease Control and Prevention. Prevention and treatment of TB among patients infected with HIV. MMWR 47(RR-20): 1-58, 1998

4a: Diagnostic Algorithm for Hypotension and/or Shock

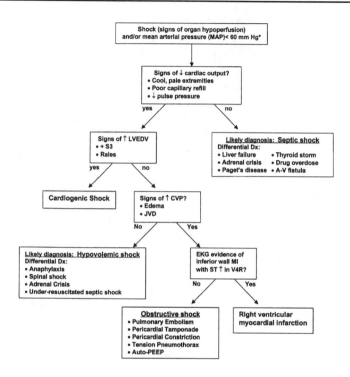

* MAP threshold is 75% of baseline value.

MAP – mean arterial pressure. LVEDV – left ventricular end diastolic volume. CVP – central venous pressure. JVD – jugular venous distension. MI – myocardial infarction. PEEP – positive end expiratory pressure.

Hall JB et al. Principles of Critical Care 2nd ed., McGraw Hill, New York, 1998

4b: Therapeutic Algorithm for Hypotension and/or Shock

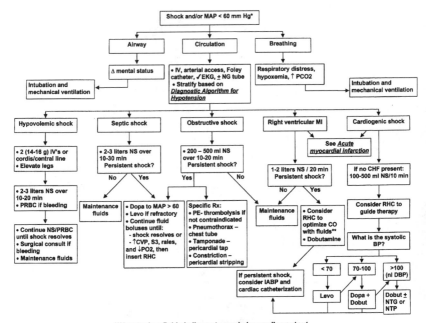

**How to do a fluid challenge to maximize cardiac output

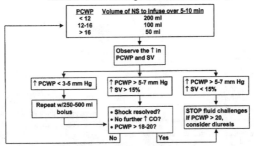

Dopa – dopamine 2-20 mcg/kg/min; Dobut – dobutamine 5-15 mcg/kg/min; Levo – levophed 2-30 mcg/kg/min; NTG – nitroglycerine 25-600 mcg/min
NTP – nitroprusside -0.1-5 mcg/kg/min. (*MAP goal is 75% of baseline value)
MAP – mean arterial pressure. DBP – diastolic blood pressure. RHC – right heart catheterization. SV – stroke volume (cardiac output/heart rate). NS – normal saline. PRBC – packed red blood cells. MI – myocardial infarction. IABP – intra-aortic balloon pump. CO – cardiac output.

Hall JB et al. Principles of Critical Care 2nd ed., McGraw Hill, New York, 1998
Guidelines for cardiopulmonary resuscitation and emergency cardiac care. JAMA 268: 2171, 1992

4c: Table of Hemodynamic Subsets

Diagnosis	CVP	PCWP	CO	SVR	Comments
Hypovolemic Shock	↓	↓	↓	↑	
Distributive Shock (Sepsis, liver failure, thyroid storm, adrenal crisis, etc.)	nl or ↓	nl or ↓	nl or ↑	↓	May present with ↓ CO if under-resuscitated
Cardiogenic Shock					
Acute MI – predominantly LV	nl	↑	↓	↑	
Acute MI – predominantly RV	↑	nl or ↓	↓	↑	
Acute mitral regurgitation	nl or ↑	↑	↓	↑	PCWP shows large V waves
Acute ventricular septal defect	nl or ↑	nl or ↑	↓*	↑	*measured CO by thermodilution or Fick method will overestimate CO if shunt is L to R. Dx by step-up in O2 sats from RA to RV. PCWP may show large V waves
Obstructive shock					
Massive pulmonary embolism	↑	nl or ↓	↓	↑	PAD >> PCWP; ↑ PVR
Pericardial tamponade	↑	↑	↓	↑	CVP ≅ PCWP; CVP shows loss of "y" descent
Tension pneumothorax	↑	↑	↓	↑	CVP ≅ PCWP
Occult autopeep	↑	↑	↓	↑	CVP ≅ PCWP. Suspect in patients with airway obstruction receiving assisted ventilation.

Normal values for hemodynamic parameters:

Central venous pressure (CVP):	2-8 mm Hg
Pulmonary capillary wedge pressure (PCWP):	5-12 mm Hg
Cardiac output (CO):	4-6 liters/min
Systemic vascular resistance (SVR):	900-1200 dyne-s/cm^5

PEEP – positive end expiratory pressure. MI – myocardial infarction. RA – right atrium. RV- right ventricle. LV – left ventricle. PAD – pulmonary artery diastolic pressure. PVR – pulmonary vascular resistance.

Hall JB et al. **Principles of Critical Care** 2nd ed., McGraw Hill, New York, 1998

4d: Hypothermia

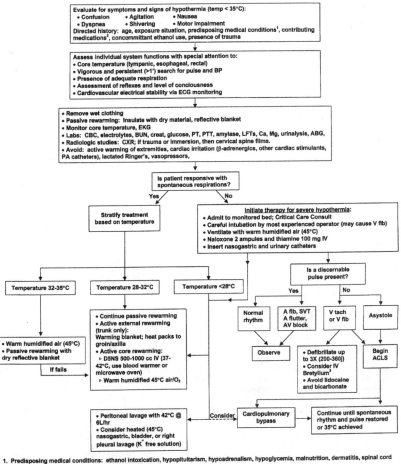

Evaluate for symptoms and signs of hypothermia (temp < 35°C):
- Confusion
- Agitation
- Nausea
- Dyspnea
- Shivering
- Motor impairment

Directed history: age, exposure situation, predisposing medical conditions[1], contributing medications[2], concommittant ethanol use, presence of trauma

Assess individual system functions with special attention to:
- Core temperature (tympanic, esophageal, rectal)
- Vigorous and persistent (>1') search for pulse and BP
- Presence of adequate respiration
- Assessment of reflexes and level of conciousness
- Cardiovascular electrical stability via ECG monitoring

- Remove wet clothing
- Passive rewarming: Insulate with dry material, reflective blanket
- Monitor core temperature, EKG
- Labs: CBC, electrolytes, BUN, creat, glucose, PT, PTT, amylase, LFTs, Ca, Mg, urinalysis, ABG,
- Radiologic studies: CXR; if trauma or immersion, then cervical spine films.
- Avoid: active warming of extremities, cardiac irritation (β-adrenergics, other cardiac stimulants, PA catheters), lactated Ringer's, vasopressors,

Is patient responsive with spontaneous respirations?

Yes → **Stratify treatment based on temperature**

No → **Initiate therapy for severe hypothermia:**
- Admit to monitored bed; Critical Care Consult
- Careful intubation by most experienced operator (may cause V fib)
- Ventilate with warm humidified air (45°C)
- Naloxone 2 ampules and thiamine 100 mg IV
- insert nasogastric and urinary catheters

Is a discernable pulse present?

Temperature 32-35°C
- Warm humidified air (45°C)
- Passive rewarming with dry reflective blanket

If fails

Temperature 28-32°C
- Continue passive rewarming
- Active external rewarming (trunk only):
  Warming blanket; heat packs to groin/axilla
- Active core rewarming:
  ▷ D5NS 500-1000 cc IV (37-42°C, use blood warmer or microwave oven)
  ▷ Warm humidified 45°C air/O₂

Temperature <28°C

Yes:
- Normal rhythm → Observe
- A fib, SVT / A flutter / AV block → Observe

No:
- V tach or V fib →
  - Defibrillate up to 3X (200-360j)
  - Consider IV Bretylium[3]
  - Avoid lidocaine and bicarbonate
- Asystole → Begin ACLS

Begin ACLS

- Peritoneal lavage with 42°C @ 6L/hr
- Consider heated (45°C) nasogastric, bladder, or right pleural lavage (K⁺ free solution)

Consider → **Cardiopulmonary bypass**

Continue until spontaneous rhythm and pulse restored or 35°C achieved

1. Predisposing medical conditions: ethanol intoxication, hypopituitarism, hypoadrenalism, hypoglycemia, malnutrition, dermatitis, spinal cord injury, diabetes, CNS lesion, sepsis, uremia, Paget's disease
2. Contributing medications: ethanol, phenothiazines, benzodiazepines, antidepressants, barbiturates, narcotics, clonidine
3. Bretylium tosylate 5-10mg/kg loading dose, 1-2 mg/min maintenance dose. Procainamide should be avoided.

Weinberg A. Hypothermia. Ann Emerg Med 22:370-377, 1993
Gentilello L. Advances in the management of hypothermia. Surg Clin NA 75:243-256, 1995
Danzi DF, Pozos RS. Accidental hypothermia. N Engl J Med 331: 1756-1760, 1994
Lazar HL. The treatment of hypothermia. N Engl J Med 337: 1545 – 47, 1997

4e: Hyperthermia

Directed Hx: Age, exposure situation (activity, temperature, humidity), predisposing factors[1], contributing medications[2], symptoms
Assess individual system functions with special attention to:
- Core temperature (tympanic, esophageal, rectal)
- Mental status examination
- Examination of skin for perspiration
- Studies: BUN, creatinine, chemistries, CBC, LFTs, pH, CPK, CXR, ECG, coagulation studies, urinalysis. Consider drug screen, salicylate level, TFTs

Consider differential diagnosis and exclude by Hx, PE, labs:

CNS Process	Drug related		Infectious dx	Other
encephalitis	lithium	malignant	typhoid fever	pheochromocytoma
status epilepticus	phencyclidine	hyperthermia (MH)[3]	tetanus	thyroid storm
meningitis	salicylate	neuroleptic malignant	sepsis	
cerebral abscess	amphetamine	syndrome (NMS)	malaria	
catatonia	anticholinergic	ETOH withdrawal		
hypothalamic infarct	cocaine	serotonin syndrome		

positive drug screen

See Toxicology algorithms and List of specific antidotes

phenothiazine or other neuroleptic

Consider NMS if rigid muscles, profuse sweating, and autonomic dysfunction present. Rx with bromocriptine 2.5-10 mg Q8H

General principles: "ABC's", ACLS if needed, D/C any offending agent
- Continous core temp monitoring
- Cooling within 1 hr = 5% mortality; cooling > 1 hr = 18% mortality
- Ice packs to neck, axillae, groin to achieve reduction of 0.1°C/min.
- Evaporative cooling by spraying room temperature water over skin and fanning. Do not use ice water or ice water baths (promotes peripheral capillary constriction and shivering, which inhibits heat loss)
- Monitor urine output for renal insufficiency
- Replete electrolytes
- Consider lorazepam 1-2 mg, diazepam 5 mg, or chlorpromazine 20-50 mg IV to suppress shivering if NMS ruled out; anti-pyretics are of little use. Dantrolene is effective in MH but has little effect in environmental heat stroke
- D5NS or 1/2 NS @150 cc/hr as guided by blood pressure, electrolytes
Avoid Ringer's lactate.

Temperature < 41°C and malaise, headache, nausea, vomiting, weakness but without coma, delirium or altered mental status

Dx: Heat Exhaustion
- Electrolyte disturbances less common
- LFT and CPK elevations are usually mild
- Continue ice packs, evaporative cooling

Discontinue cooling measures once core temperature < 39°C

Treat rhabdomyolysis with:
- Mannitol 12.5 g IV
- ↑ IV fluids: 2 ampules of Na bicarbonate in 1 liter of 1/2NS or D51/2NS at 200 cc/hr

rhabdomyolysis present

Temperature > 40°C + any altered mental status (coma, delirium, seizures) + heat exposure
Sweating usually (but not invariably) absent.

Dx: Heat Stroke
- Treat electrolyte disturbances: hyponatremia, hypocalcemia, hypo- or hyperglycemia commonly seen
- LFT elevations are usually transient; if persistent and high, consider GI consult
- R/O infection (up to 50% in one series)

Utilize evaporative cooling unit if available by suspending naked patient on net over drainage table while skin is sprayed with 15°C water and fanned with 48°C air; usually reduces cooling time to 1 H. Otherwise, continue ice packs and evaporative cooling.

Consider peritoneal lavage with 2L 6°C dialysate over 20 minutes

1. Predisposing factors: extremes of age, dehydration, gastroenteritis, occupational exposure, athletic activity, obesity, hyperthyroidism
2. Contributing medications: anticholinergics, lithium, atropine, antihistamines, anti-depressants, phenothiazines, β-blockers, amphetamines, phencyclidine, cocaine, diuretics
3. Rare; occurs within 11 hours of inhalational anesthetics or depolarizing muscle relaxants. Sx: muscle rigidity, hypotension, tachycardia, arrhythmias, acidosis, hyperkalemia, cyanosis, rhabdomyolysis and DIC. Rx: Dantrolene sodium 1 mg/kg, increase prn to max of 10 mg/kg then 1-2 mg/kg Q6 for 1-3 days

Simon H. Hyperthermia. N Engl J Med 329:483-487, 1993   Harchelroad F. Acute thermoregulatory disorders. Clin Geriat Med 9: 621-639, 1993
Bouchama A. Heatstroke: A new look at an ancient disease. Int Care Med 21: 623-5, 1995
Yaqub B, Aldeeb S. Heatstroke: aetiopathogenesis, neurological characteristics, treatment and outcome. J Neurol Sci 136: 144-51, 1998

4f: Alcohol Withdrawal and Delirium Tremens

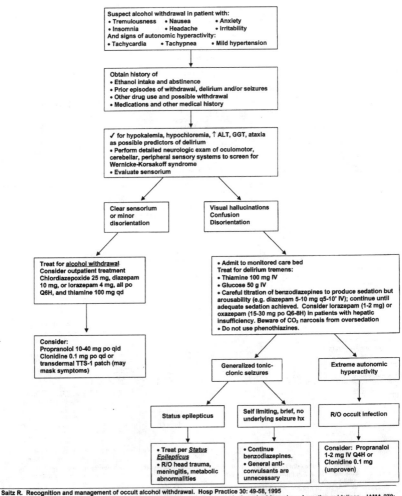

Suspect alcohol withdrawal in patient with:
- Tremulousness
- Nausea
- Anxiety
- Insomnia
- Headache
- Irritability

And signs of autonomic hyperactivity:
- Tachycardia
- Tachypnea
- Mild hypertension

↓

Obtain history of
- Ethanol intake and abstinence
- Prior episodes of withdrawal, delirium and/or seizures
- Other drug use and possible withdrawal
- Medications and other medical history

↓

- ✓ for hypokalemia, hypochloremia, ↑ ALT, GGT, ataxia as possible predictors of delirium
- Perform detailed neurologic exam of oculomotor, cerebellar, peripheral sensory systems to screen for Wernicke-Korsakoff syndrome
- Evaluate sensorium

Clear sensorium or minor disorientation

Visual hallucinations Confusion Disorientation

Treat for <u>alcohol withdrawal</u>
Consider outpatient treatment
Chlordiazepoxide 25 mg, diazepam 10 mg, or lorazepam 4 mg, all po Q6H, and thiamine 100 mg qd

↓

Consider:
Propranolol 10-40 mg po qid
Clonidine 0.1 mg po qd or transdermal TTS-1 patch (may mask symptoms)

- Admit to monitored care bed
Treat for delirium tremens:
- Thiamine 100 mg IV
- Glucose 50 g IV
- Careful titration of benzodiazepines to produce sedation but arousability (e.g. diazepam 5-10 mg q5-10' IV); continue until adequate sedation achieved. Consider lorazepam (1-2 mg) or oxazepam (15-30 mg po Q6-8H) in patients with hepatic insufficiency. Beware of CO_2 narcosis from oversedation
- Do not use phenothiazines.

Generalized tonic-clonic seizures

Extreme autonomic hyperactivity

Status epilepticus

Self limiting, brief, no underlying seizure hx

R/O occult infection

- Treat per *Status Epilepticus*
- R/O head trauma, meningitis, metabolic abnormalities

- Continue benzodiazepines.
- General anti-convulsants are unnecessary

Consider: Propranolol 1-2 mg IV Q4H or Clonidine 0.1 mg (unproven)

Saitz R. Recognition and management of occult alcohol withdrawal. Hosp Practice 30: 49-58, 1995
Mayo-Smith M. Pharmacological management of alcohol withdrawal: A meta-analysis and evidence based practice guidelines. JAMA 278: 144-51, 1997
Hall W, Zador D. The alcohol withdrawal syndrome. Lancet 349: 1897 – 1900, 1997

4g: Equations

Conversions

Weight:

1kg = 2.2 lbs	1 lb = 0.454 kg	1 ounce = 30 g
1 tspn = 5 ml	1 tbspn = 15 ml	1 ounce = 30 ml

Temperature

$$°F = 32 + 9/5(°C) \qquad °C = 5/9(°F - 32)$$

1 inch = 2.54 cm   1 cm = 0.3973 inch

$BSA (m^2) = [(ht(cm) \times wt(kg))/3600]^{0.5}$

Ventilation

$PAO_2 = FIO_2(Pb-47) - PCO_2/R$
age correction for "normal" $O_2 = 100 - 1/3$ (age)
$PACO_2 = (0.863 \times VCO_2)/V_A$
Oxygen content (C) = $(1.36 \times Hb \times \%Sat) + 0.003(PO_2)$
$Qs/Qt = [(Cc'O_2 - CaO_2)/(Cc'O_2 - CvO_2)] \times 100$
Qs/Qt estimate: (A-a gradient on 100%)/16

Compliance = $VT/(Pplateau - peep)$

Resistance = $60 \times (Ppleak - Pplateau)$ /Flow

$V_D/V_T = (PaCO_2 - PeCO_2)/PaCO_2$

P - partial pressure (A - alveolar, a - arterial, e - mixed expired); FIO2 - fraction of inspired O2; R - respiratory exchange ratio (≈0.8); V_A - minute alveolar ventilation; V_D/V_T - dead space /tidal volume ratio; c' - end capillary, v - mixed venous

Hemodynamics

Mean arterial pressure (MAP) = (1/3)systolic + (2/3)diastolic
Fick equation: Cardiac output (CO) = $10 \times VO_2/CaO_2 - CvO_2$
Systemic vascular resistance (SVR) = $[(MAP - mRAP) \times 80]/CO$
Pulmonary vascular resistance (PVR) = $[(mPAP - PCW) \times 80]/CO$
Oxygen delivery (DO2) = $CO \times 1.36 \times Hb \times SaO_2$
Cerebral Perfusion Pressure = MAP - ICP

mRAP - mean right atrial pressure; mPAP - mean pulmonary artery pressure; PCW - pulmonary artery occlusion pressure ICP - intracranial pressure

Acid Base Disorders (See *Renal* section)

Acute respiratory acidosis:	$\Delta pH = 0.008(\Delta PCO_2)$
Chronic respiratory acidosis:	$\Delta pH = 0.003(\Delta PCO_2)$
Acute respiratory alkalosis:	$\Delta pH = 0.008(\Delta PCO_2)$
Chronic respiratory alkalosis:	$\Delta pH = 0.002(\Delta PCO_2)$

Anion gap = Na - (Cl + HCO3)   Normal < 12-15; AG will decrease by 2.5 for every 1 g/dl decrease in albumin

Nutrition (see *Nutrition equations* and *Nutrition* section)

Harris - Benedict equations: Males: REE = 66.47 + 13.75(IBW) + 5.0H - 6.76A
                                               Females: REE = 655.1 + 9.5(IBW) + 9.56H - 4.68A
Sherman equation   MEE = $9.27 (P_ECO_2)(V_E)$
Ligget - St. John - LeFrak equation   MEE = $95.18 (CO) (Hb) (SaO_2 - SvO_2)$
Nitrogen balance   Nitrogen balance = Protein intake(g)/6.25 - (24 hr UUN(g) + 4)

REE – resting energy expenditure. MEE – measured energy expenditure. IBW – ideal body weight (kg). H – height (cm).
A – age (years). CO – cardiac output. VE – minute ventilation. UUN – urinary urea nitrogen

Renal/Fluid and electrolytes

Total body water = 0.6 X lean body weight (kg) (males); = 0.5 X lean body weight (kg) (females)
Estimation of lean/ideal body weight: females: =45.5 kg for first 5', then 2.3 kg each additional inch
                                                             males: =48 kg for first 5', then 2.7 kg each additional inch
Creatinine clearance (CCL) = (urine Cr (mg/dl) X total volume (ml)/[serum Cr (mg/dl)X time(min)]
Cockcroft-Gault formula : CCL = [(140-age) X weight(kg)/72 X serum Cr] X (0.85 if female, obese, or edema)
Cl⁻ deficit = 0.5(wt in kg)(103-serum Cl⁻(meq))
Na deficit = 0.6 (wt in kg)(140 - Na)+ 140(H_2O deficit in l)
H_2O deficit = 0.6 (wt in kg)(Na/140 - 1)
Calculated osmolality = 2(Na) + (glucose/18) + (BUN/2.8) + (mannitol/18) + (EtOH/4.6)
Osmolar gap = actual osmolality - calculated. Normal range: 0-5.
FeNa = (Urine Na/Plasma Na)/(Urine Creatinine/Plasma Creatinine). FeNa < 1 is prerenal
Na correction for high glucose: Actual Na = measured Na + 1.6 X [(measured glucose - 100)/100]
Ca correction for low albumin: Corrected Ca = measured Ca + 0.8 (normal albumin - measured albumin)

Cr – creatinine.

4h: Ventilator Management

Indications for mechanical ventilation

Hypoxemia	Hypercapnia	Clinical
pO2 < 55 torr or SO2 < 92% despite supplemental oxygen delivery.	pCO2 > 44 torr acutely; or pCO2 elevated chronically with pH < 7.25 despite non-invasive ventilation assist devices.	Respiratory distress accompanied by shock or somnolence

Physician Orders:
Intubate patient: Oral ET tube size ≥ 7.0 (in adults) to avoid high airway resistance, suctioning difficulty, and possible occlusion from mucus and blood.

Initial Ventilator Settings:

Mode	Assist/Control (A/C*) or Intermittent Mandatory Ventilation (IMV*):
Inspired Oxygen (FIO2)	Select FIO2 based on PaO2 from previous ABG, or empirically start at FIO2 = 1.0 and decrease until SO2 = 94% (paO2 approximately 75 torr).
PEEP (cmH2O)	Begin at 5 to provide physiologic backpressure lost by the ET tube bypassing glottal muscles. Increase PEEP in increments of 2.5 to PEEP maximum* if the FIO2 ≥ 0.6.
Respiratory Rate (RR)	Begin at 8 - 12. Increase the RR if the patient's spontaneous RR > 6 above the set RR.
Tidal Volume (VT)	Begin at 8 or 10 mL/kg and round off to the nearest 50 mL. Consider lower VT (5-10 ml/kg) in ARDS.
Nebulizer treatments	Albuterol, ipratropium bromide when indicated, frequency: at least q4h. See _COPD acute respiratory failure_ Consider 2% bicarbonate solutions as broncholytic.

Physician orders to adjust ventilator after initial settings and ABG:

Oxygenation (PO₂)	Ventilation (PCO₂)
Adjust FIO2 and PEEP to alter SaO2. ↓ The SaO2 varies directly with the FIO2 and PEEP. ↓ For hypoxemia (SaO2 < 94%) requiring FIO2 > 0.6, first increase PEEP in steps of 2.5 to a PEEP maximum* above 5. ↓ If hypoxemia persists, then increase the FIO2 in steps of 0.10 until 1.0 is reached or SO2>93%. ↓ For SO2 > 95% at PEEP maximum*, FIO2 is first reduced in steps of 0.10 until < 0.6, then PEEP is reduced in steps of 2.5 to a minimum of 5 before further reductions of FIO2.	Adjust RR and VT to alter pCO2 and pH. ↓ The pCO2 varies inversely with the VE* (RR x VT) ↓ If pH < 7.35, increase VE (to lower pCO2) by increasing RR by 2 to a maximum of 24; if acidemia persists, consider increasing VT in steps of 50 mL to maximum of 15mL/kg with the following caveats: • In ARDS, high VT may cause alveolar damage; Limit VT to keep plateau pressure ≤ 35 and allow permissive CO2 retention and lower pH. • In COPD or asthma, high VE may cause autopeep. Autopeep should be measured before increasing VE. Aim for pH ~7.35, not for normal PCO2; minimize autopeep; keep plateau pressure < 30 and allow permissive CO2 retention. ↓ If pH > 7.45, decrease VE (to raise pCO2) by decreasing RR by 2 until ≤ 8, then decrease VT in steps of 50 mL. If patient's RR remains elevated despite the ventilator RR reduction, consider sedation.

Pulmonary consultation should be considered for any patient on a ventilator and should be obtained for patients with ARDS or ventilatory failure due to any primary pulmonary disease state.

*Definitions:
A/C: Patient receives a set volume for every breath triggered by either patient effort (assist), or by time (control, based on the set Respiratory Rate).
IMV: Patient receives a set volume for the set Respiratory Rate, additional spontaneous breaths (non-set volume) can be taken at any time.
PEEP maximum: Positive End Expiratory Pressure (PEEP) producing improved oxygenation without significant compromise in hemodynamics, such as cardiac output, mixed venous saturation, and BP.
VE: Minute ventilation = Respiratory Rate x Tidal Volume
SaO2: Arterial oxygen saturation

Branson RD. Monitoring ventilator function. Crit Care Clin 11:127-143, 1995.
Tobin MJ. Mechanical ventilation. N Engl J Med 330:1056-1061, 1994.
Hinson JR, Marini JJ. Principles of mechanical ventilator use in respiratory failure. Ann Rev Med 43:341-361, 1992.

4i: Management of Hypertensive Emergencies

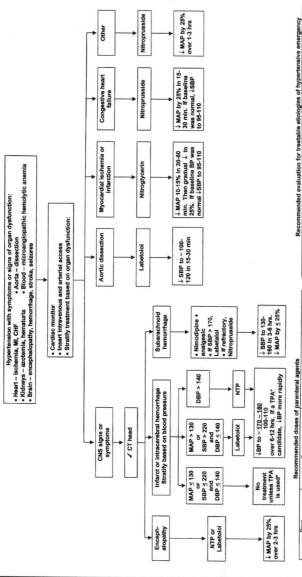

Hypertension with symptoms or signs of organ dysfunction:
- Heart – ischemia, MI, CHF
- Aorta – dissection
- Kidneys – azotemia, hematuria
- Blood – microangiopathic hemolytic anemia
- Brain – encephalopathy, hemorrhage, stroke, seizures

- Cardiac monitor
- Insert intravenous and arterial access
- Stratify treatment based on organ dysfunction:

Aortic dissection → Labetolol → ↓ SBP to ~100-120 in 15-30 min

Myocardial ischemia or Infarction → Nitroglycerin → ↓ MAP 10-15% in 30-60 min. Then gradual ↓ to 25%. If baseline BP was normal ↓SBP to 95-110

Congestive heart failure → Nitroprusside → ↓ MAP by 25% in 15-30 min. If baseline was normal, ↓SBP to 95-110

Other → Nitroprusside → ↓ MAP by 25% over 1-3 hrs

CNS signs or symptoms → ✓ CT head

Encephalopathy → NTP or Labetolol → ↓ MAP by 25% over 2-3 hrs

Infarct or intracerebral hemorrhage Stratify based on blood pressure

- MAP ≤ 130 or SBP ≤ 220 and DBP ≤ 140 → No treatment unless TPA is used*
- MAP > 130 or SBP > 220 and DBP ≤ 140 → Labetolol
- DBP > 140 → NTP

→ ↓BP to 170 – 180 / 100-110 over 6-12 hrs. If a TPA* candidate, ↓BP more rapidly

Subarachnoid hemorrhage
- Nimodipine + analgesic
- If SBP > 170, Labetolol
- If refractory, Nitroprusside

→ ↓ SBP to 130-160 in 3-6 hrs. ↓ MAP by ≤ 25%

Recommended doses of parenteral agents

Drug	Dose	Titration
Nitroprusside (NTP)	0.25 – 10 mcg/kg/min	↑ 0.5 – 1.0 mcg/kg/min q 3-5 min
Nitroglycerine (NTG)	5-600 mcg/min	↑ 5-10 mcg/min q 3–5 min
Labetolol	10-80 mg bolus; 0.5-2 mg /min infusion	Give 10-20 mg bolus q 10 min; can ↑ to 40-80 mg q10 min up to 300 mg
Nimodipine	60 mg po q4h X 21 days	

Recommended evaluation for treatable etiologies of hypertensive emergency

Diagnosis	Evaluation
Renovascular hypertension	High index of suspicion: IA digital subtraction angiogram Moderate suspicion: MR angilogram, Spiral CT or Duplex US
Pheochromocytoma	24 hr urine for VMA / metanephrine. If positive → localize by CT/MRI. If negative, →[131]I-monoiodobenzylguanidine scan

CNS – central nervous system. CT – computerized tomography. MI – myocardial infarction. MAP – mean arterial pressure. SAP – systolic blood pressure. DBP – diastolic blood pressure.

Gifford RW. Management of hypertensive crisis. JAMA 266: 829, 1991

Adams HA et al. Guidelines for the management of patients with acute ischemic stroke. Stroke 25: 1901, 1994

Brandt T et al. Neurologic Disorders: Course and Treatment, Academic Press, 1996

* See *Acute Stroke* for TPA (tissue plasminogen activator) indications

5a: Dysphagia

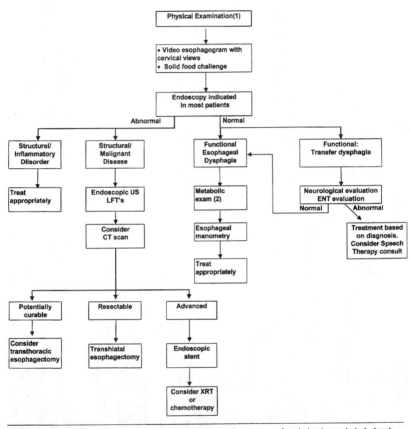

(1) Physical exam: Should include detailed orophayngeal, head and neck exam, exam of cervical and supraclavicular lymph nodes, and a detailed neurologic exam with focus on cranial nerves, speech and frontal release signs.

(2) Metabolic screen: includes sed rate, polymyositis, SCL-70 (scleroderma), anti-centromere antibody (CREST), ANA (SLE), fasting glucose, thyroid studies (myxedma). Consider biopsy for amyloidosis during endoscopy.

5b: Management of Peptic Ulcer Disease

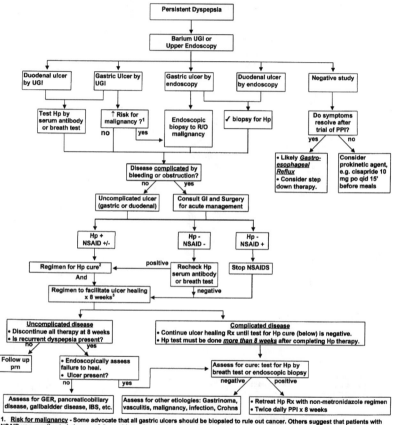

Persistent Dyspepsia

Barium UGI or Upper Endoscopy

- **Duodenal ulcer by UGI**
- **Gastric Ulcer by UGI**
- **Gastric ulcer by endoscopy**
- **Duodenal ulcer by endoscopy**
- **Negative study**

Test Hp by serum antibody or breath test

↑ Risk for malignancy ?[1] — no / yes

Endoscopic biopsy to R/O malignancy

✓ biopsy for Hp

Do symptoms resolve after trial of PPI? — yes / no

- yes: • Likely *Gastro-esophageal Reflux* • Consider step down therapy.
- no: Consider prokinetic agent, e.g. cisapride 10 mg po qid 15' before meals

Disease complicated by bleeding or obstruction? — no / yes

- no: **Uncomplicated ulcer (gastric or duodenal)**
- yes: **Consult GI and Surgery for acute management**

- **Hp + NSAID +/-**
- **Hp - NSAID -**
- **Hp - NSAID +**

Regimen for Hp cure[2] ← positive — **Recheck Hp serum antibody or breath test** — negative → / **Stop NSAIDS**

And

Regimen to facilitate ulcer healing x 8 weeks[3]

Uncomplicated disease
- Discontinue all therapy at 8 weeks
- Is recurrent dyspepsia present? — no / yes
  - no: **Follow up prn**
  - yes: • Endoscopically assess failure to heal. • Ulcer present? — no / yes

Complicated disease
- Continue ulcer healing Rx until test for Hp cure (below) is negative.
- Hp test must be done *more than 8 weeks* after completing Hp therapy.

Assess for cure: test for Hp by breath test or endoscopic biopsy — negative / positive

- no: **Assess for GER, pancreaticobiliary disease, gallbladder disease, IBS, etc.**
- yes: **Assess for other etiologies: Gastrinoma, vasculitis, malignancy, infection, Crohns**
- negative:
- positive: • Retreat Hp Rx with non-metronidazole regimen • Twice daily PPI x 8 weeks

1. **Risk for malignancy** - Some advocate that all gastric ulcers should be biopsied to rule out cancer. Others suggest that patients with NSAID use, small antral ulcers , < 0.5 cm with regular margins and without nodularity or mass effect may be treated as a benign ulcer without endoscopy. These patients should have complete ulcer healing documented by repeat barium study.

2. **Regimens for Hp cure** (This is not a complete list. Regimens change rapidly and current regimens should be sought)
- Metronidazole 250 mg PO QID, Tetracycline 500 mg PO QID, Bismuth subsalicylate 2 tablets PO QID, Ranitidine 150 mg bid (14 day) OR
- Metronidazole 500 mg PO BID, Clarithromycin 500 mg PO BID, Omeprazole 20 mg PO BID (7 day) OR
- Amoxacillin 1000 mg PO BID, Clarithromycin 500 mg PO BID, Omeprazole 20 mg PO BID (7 day) OR
- Tritec (ranitidine/ bismuth combination) bid, metronidazole 500 mg bid, clarithromycin 500 mg bid (7 day)

3. **Regimens to facilitate ulcer healing**
Proton pump inhibitor: Omeprazole 20 mg PO QD, Lansoprazole 30 mg PO QD
H2 receptor antagonist: Cimetidine 400 mg PO BID, Ranitidine 150 mg PO BID, Famotidine 20 mg PO BID, Nizatidine 150 mg PO BID
Other: Sucralfate 1 gram PO QID

Abbreviations: Hp = Helicobacter pylori, NSAID = Non-steroidal anti-inflammatory drug, IBS = irritable bowel syndrome
Soll, A. H. Medical treatment of Peptic Ulcer Disease: Practice guidelines. JAMA; 275:622 1996
Isenberg, J.I. et al. Acid-Peptic Disorders. In Textbook of Gastroenterology, 2nd edition. T.Yamada ed. Lippincott Co., Philadelphia. 1996.
Freston, J.W. Emerging strategies for managing peptic ulcer disease.. Scand J Gastroenterol. 29(S201):49 1994

5c: Gastroesophageal Reflux

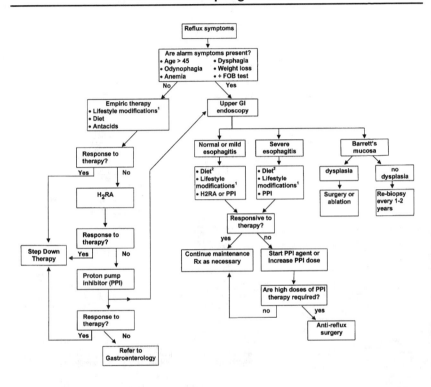

[Reflux symptoms]

[Are alarm symptoms present?
• Age > 45   • Dysphagia
• Odynophagia   • Weight loss
• Anemia   • + FOB test]
No / Yes

No →
[Empiric therapy
• Lifestyle modifications[1]
• Diet
• Antacids]

Yes →
[Upper GI endoscopy]

[Response to therapy?]
Yes / No

[Normal or mild esophagitis]
• Diet[2]
• Lifestyle modifications[1]
• H2RA or PPI

[Severe esophagitis]
• Diet[2]
• Lifestyle modifications[1]
• PPI

[Barrett's mucosa]
[dysplasia] → [Surgery or ablation]
[no dysplasia] → [Re-biopsy every 1-2 years]

[H2RA]

[Response to therapy?]
Yes / No

[Step Down Therapy]

[Responsive to therapy?]
yes / no

[Continue maintenance Rx as necessary]

[Start PPI agent or Increase PPI dose]

[Proton pump inhibitor (PPI)]

[Response to therapy?]
Yes / No

[Are high doses of PPI therapy required?]
no / yes

[Anti-reflux surgery]

[Refer to Gastroenterology]

[1]Lifestyle modification:
- Do not lie down for 2 hours post prandial
- Elevate head of bed 4 to 6 inches
- Stop smoking

[2]Diet   Avoid fatty foods, eating late, large meals

FOB – fecal occult blood
H2RA -- Histamine-2 receptor blockers:
   cimetidine 300 mg po bid or famotidine 20 mg bid or nizatadine 150 mg po bid or ranitidine 150 mg po bid
PPI -- Protein pump inhibitors:
   Omeprazole 20 mg po qd or Lansoprazole 30 mg po qd before eating

Spechler SJ. Barrett's Esophagus. The Gastroenterologist, 1994: 2: 273-84
Kimmig JM. Treatment and prevention of relapse of mild oesophagitis with omeprazole and cisapride: Comparison of two strategies. Aliment Pharmacol Ther 1995; 9:281-286
Devault KR. Current Management of gastroesophageal reflux disease. The Gastroenterologist 1996; 4: 24-32

5d: Approach to the Patient with Acute Diarrhea

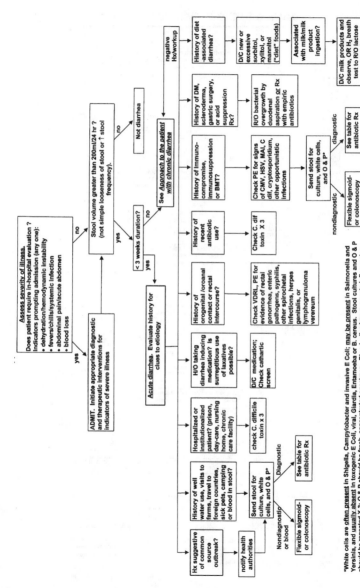

*White cells are often present in Shigella, Campylobacter and invasive E Coli; may be present in Salmonella and Yersinia, and usually absent in toxigenic E Coli, viral, Giardia, Entamoeba or B. cereus. Stool cultures and O & P should be repeated X 3; O & P should be fresh, concentrated specimen. Bloody diarrhea suggests inflammatory bowel disease, Salmonella, Shigella, Campylobacter, Yersinia, E Coli, Entamoeba, C diff, or ischemia. O & P - Ova and Parasites. C. dif - Clostridia difficile, BMT - bone marrow transplant, CMV - cytomegalovirus, HSV - herpes simplex virus, MAI - mycobacterium avium-intracellulare

5e: Approach to the Patient with Chronic Diarrhea

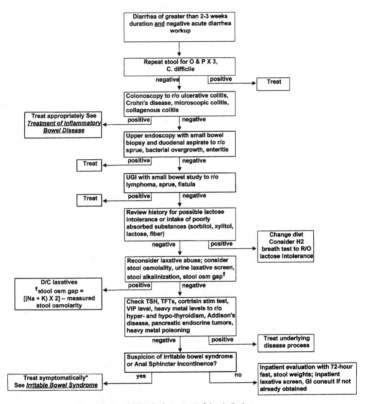

Diarrhea of greater than 2-3 weeks duration and negative acute diarrhea workup

↓

Repeat stool for O & P X 3, C. difficile
- negative
- positive → **Treat**

↓

Colonoscopy to r/o ulcerative colitis, Crohn's disease, microscopic colitis, collagenous colitis
- positive → **Treat appropriately See *Treatment of Inflammatory Bowel Disease***
- negative

↓

Upper endoscopy with small bowel biopsy and duodenal aspirate to r/o sprue, bacterial overgrowth, enteritis
- positive → **Treat**
- negative

↓

UGI with small bowel study to r/o lymphoma, sprue, fistula
- positive → **Treat**
- negative

↓

Review history for possible lactose intolerance or intake of poorly absorbed substances (sorbitol, xylitol, lactose, fiber)
- negative
- positive → **Change diet Consider H2 breath test to R/O lactose intolerance**

↓

Reconsider laxative abuse; consider stool osmolality, urine laxative screen, stool alkalinization, stool osm gap[†]
- positive → **D/C laxatives** [†]stool osm gap = [[(Na + K) X 2] – measured stool osmolarity
- negative

↓

Check TSH, TFTs, cortrisin stim test, VIP level, heavy metal levels to r/o hyper- and hypo-thyroidism, Addison's disease, pancreatic endocrine tumors, heavy metal poisoning
- negative
- positive → **Treat underlying disease process**

↓

Suspicion of Irritable bowel syndrome or Anal Sphincter Incontinence?
- yes → **Treat symptomatically* See *Irritable Bowel Syndrome***
- no → **Inpatient evaluation with 72-hour fast, stool weights; inpatient laxative screen, GI consult if not already obtained**

*Some symptomatic therapies for treatment of chronic diarrhea

Class	Drug	Dose
Antisecretory	Bismuth subsalicylate	2 tabs every 30-60 minutes to maximum of 8 doses/24 hours
Adsorbent	Attapulgite (Donnagel, Kaopectate, Parepectolin Diasorb)	As directed
Opiates	Lomotil(diphenoxylate/ atropine) Imodium(loperamide) Tincture of opium	up to 2 tabs qid 4mg(2tabs) 3-6 drops q 6 hours
Adrenergic blockers	clonidine	0.1 mg - 0.3 mg po q 8 hours

Donowitz M Kokke FT Saidi R. Evaluation of patients with chronic diarrhea. New England Journal of Medicine 332(11):725-9, 1995.
Powell DS Approach to the patient with diarrhea. In: Yamada T, ed. Textbook of gastroenterology. Philadelphia: J.B. Lippincott, 1995: 813-831.
Fine KD Krejs GJ Fordtran JS. Diarrhea. In: Sleisenger MH, Fordtran JS, eds. Gastrointestinal disease: pathophysiology, diagnosis, management.. 5th ed. Vol. 2. Philadelphia: S.B. Saunders, 1993: 1043-1072.

5f: Constipation

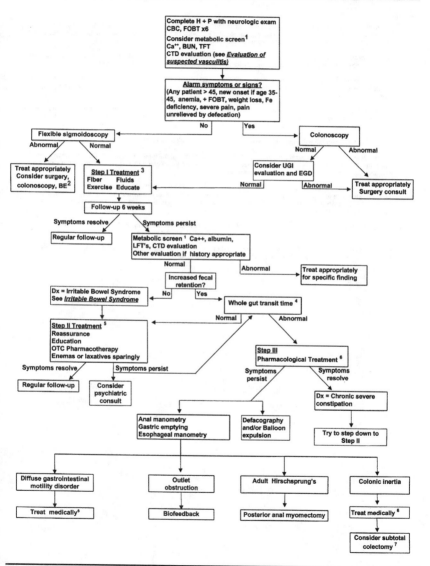

Complete H + P with neurologic exam
CBC, FOBT x6

Consider metabolic screen[1]
Ca++, BUN, TFT
CTD evaluation (see *Evaluation of suspected vasculitis*)

Alarm symptoms or signs?
(Any patient > 45, new onset if age 35-45, anemia, + FOBT, weight loss, Fe deficiency, severe pain, pain unrelieved by defecation)

No → Flexible sigmoidoscopy

Yes → Colonoscopy

Flexible sigmoidoscopy:
- Abnormal → Treat appropriately Consider surgery, colonoscopy, BE[2]
- Normal → **Step I Treatment**[3] Fiber Fluids Exercise Educate

Colonoscopy:
- Normal → Consider UGI evaluation and EGD
- Abnormal → Treat appropriately Surgery consult

Consider UGI evaluation and EGD:
- Normal
- Abnormal → Treat appropriately Surgery consult

Follow-up 6 weeks

Symptoms resolve → Regular follow-up

Symptoms persist → Metabolic screen[1] Ca++, albumin, LFT's, CTD evaluation Other evaluation if history appropriate

- Normal → Increased fecal retention?
- Abnormal → Treat appropriately for specific finding

Increased fecal retention?
- No → Dx = Irritable Bowel Syndrome See *Irritable Bowel Syndrome*
- Yes → Whole gut transit time[4]

Dx = Irritable Bowel Syndrome → **Step II Treatment**[5] Reassurance Education OTC Pharmacotherapy Enemas or laxatives sparingly

Whole gut transit time[4]:
- Normal
- Abnormal → **Step III Pharmacological Treatment**[6]

Step II Treatment:
- Symptoms resolve → Regular follow-up
- Symptoms persist → Consider psychiatric consult

Step III Pharmacological Treatment[6]:
- Symptoms persist
- Symptoms resolve → Dx = Chronic severe constipation → Try to step down to Step II

Symptoms persist:
- Anal manometry Gastric emptying Esophageal manometry
- Defacography and/or Balloon expulsion

Diffuse gastrointestinal motility disorder → Treat medically[8]

Outlet obstruction → Biofeedback

Adult Hirschsprung's → Posterior anal myomectomy

Colonic inertia → Treat medically[6] → Consider subtotal colectomy[7]

55

5f: Constipation (continued)

1. Metabolic screen should include: fasting glucose, thyroid function, calcium and electrolytes. In selected patients , evaluation of CTD, serologies (see *Evaluation of suspected vasculitis* and *Interpretation of positive fluoresent antinuclear antibody test* algorithms), amylase, heavy metal poisoning, especially lead, should be considered.

2. Barium enema is most useful in the evaluation of extrinsic lesions, rectocele or rectal prolapse, endometriosis, extrinsic neoplasm (ovarian, prostate, renal, mesenteric, lymphoma), severe stricture or large uterine fibroid.

3. Step I: Non-pharmacologic treatment: Stop aggravating medications, 25-30 gram high-fiber diet, exercise, fluids, bowel retraining, and patient education. Often useful to initiate these treatments after bowel cleansing with tap water enemas o r osmotic laxatives.

4. Whole Gut Transit Time: Several techniques available. Least expensive, which is also highly effective, is the radio-paque marker study. Patient swallows 20 radio-opaque plastic markers. Abdominal x-ray (KUB) is taken 3 hours and 4 days later.80% of markers should be eliminated after 4 days. If markers are present, another x-ray on day 7 may be useful.

5. Step II: Non-prescription therapy: If constipation persists, over-the-counter laxatives should be added to Step I treatment.
Emphasis should be on minimizing the use of contact laxatives. Osmotic, magnesium based salts are safe when used sparingly. They cannot be used in patient s with renal failure. Intermittent perging with contact laxatives or tap water enemas may prevent excessive distention of bowel loops.

6. Step III: Pharmacologic Treatment:: Should emphasize safety, low cost and efficacy. Osmotiic laxative including Milk of Magneisa, saline or balanced PEG solutions. Avoid habitual use of laxatives or enemas, although their judicious use is helpful. Avoid agents that increase bloating/gas: carbonated beverages, gaseous foods, poorly absorbed carbohydrates (lactulose, sorbitol, lactose).

7. Subtotal Colectomy: Recommended in highly selected patients who have normal upper GI motility and normal psychological status. Procedure of choice is a subtotal colectomy, ileo-rectal anastomosis. Very rarely necessary.

FOBT - fecal occult blood test; CTD – connective tissue disease, PEG - polyethylene glycol (e.g. Colyte, Golytely, Nulytiely; 4-8 oz QOD, increase as needed. Some authors recommend 1 liter Q week.

5g: Irritable Bowel Syndrome

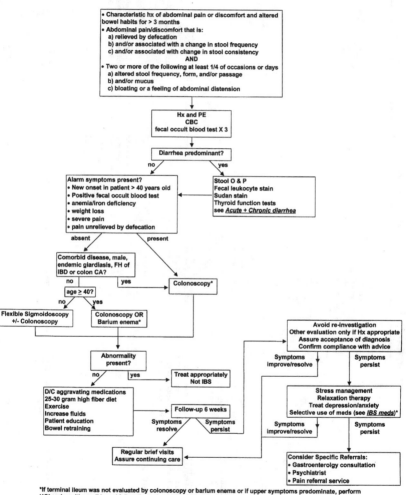

• Characteristic hx of abdominal pain or discomfort and altered bowel habits for > 3 months
• Abdominal pain/discomfort that is:
  a) relieved by defecation
  b) and/or associated with a change in stool frequency
  c) and/or associated with change in stool consistency
                        AND
• Two or more of the following at least 1/4 of occasions or days
  a) altered stool frequency, form, and/or passage
  b) and/or mucus
  c) bloating or a feeling of abdominal distension

Hx and PE
CBC
fecal occult blood test X 3

Diarrhea predominant?

no / yes

Alarm symptoms present?
• New onset in patient > 40 years old
• Positive fecal occult blood test
• anemia/iron deficiency
• weight loss
• severe pain
• pain unrelieved by defecation

Stool O & P
Fecal leukocyte stain
Sudan stain
Thyroid function tests
see *Acute + Chronic diarrhea*

absent / present

Comorbid disease, male, endemic giardiasis, FH of IBD or colon CA?

no / yes

age ≥ 40?

Colonoscopy*

no / yes

Flexible Sigmoidoscopy +/- Colonoscopy

Colonoscopy OR Barium enema*

Avoid re-investigation
Other evaluation only if Hx appropriate
Assure acceptance of diagnosis
Confirm compliance with advice

Abnormality present?

Symptoms improve/resolve   Symptoms persist

no / yes

Treat appropriately
Not IBS

D/C aggravating medications
25-30 gram high fiber diet
Exercise
Increase fluids
Patient education
Bowel retraining

Follow-up 6 weeks

Stress management
Relaxation therapy
Treat depression/anxiety
Selective use of meds (see *IBS meds*)*

Symptoms resolve   Symptoms persist

Symptoms improve/resolve   Symptoms persist

Regular brief visits
Assure continuing care

Consider Specific Referrals:
• Gastroenterology consultation
• Psychiatrist
• Pain referral service

*If terminal ileum was not evaluated by colonoscopy or barium enema or if upper symptoms predominate, perform UGI series with small bowel follow through or enterclysis examination
IBD: inflammatory bowel disease. Ca: cancer. IBS: Irritable bowel syndrome. FH: Family history

Longstreth GF. Irritable bowel syndrome. Diagnosis in the managed care era. Dig Dis Sci 1997; 42:1105-11
Farthing MJ. Irritable bowel, irritable body, or irritable brain? BMJ 310; 1995: 171-5

5h: Irritable Bowel Syndrome Medications

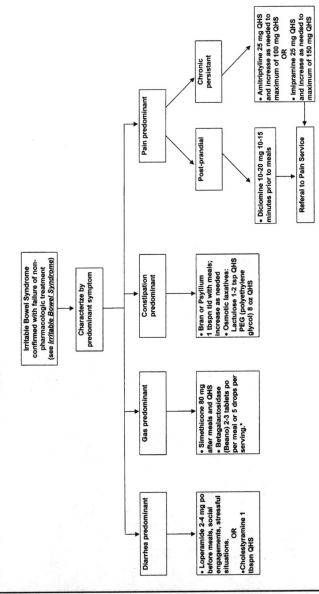

Irritable Bowel Syndrome confirmed with failure of non-pharmacologic treatment (see *Irritable Bowel Syndrome*)

Charcterize by predominant symptom

Diarrhea predominant
- Loperamide 2-4 mg po before meals, social engagements, stressful situations.
  OR
- Cholestyramine 1 tbspn QHS

Gas predominant
- Simethicone 80 mg after meals and QHS
- Betagalactosidase (Beano) 2-3 tablets po per meal or 5 drops per serving.*

Constipation predominant
- Bran or Psyllium 1 tbspn tid with meals; increase as needed
- Osmotic laxatives: Lactulose 1-2 tsp QHS PEG (polyethylene glycol) 8 oz QHS

Pain predominant

Post-prandial
- Diciomine 10-20 mg 10-15 minutes prior to meals

Chronic persistant
- Amitriptyline 25 mg QHS and increase as needed to maximum of 100 mg QHS
  OR
- Imipramine 25 mg QHS and increase as needed to maximum of 150 mg QHS

Referal to Pain Service

*Effective in foods containing the sugars raffinose, stachyose, and/or verboscose found in oats, legumes and cruciferous vegetables.

5i: Clinical Approach to Acute Pancreatitis

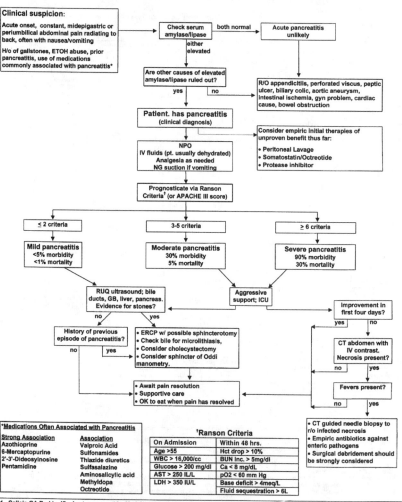

Clinical suspicion:

Acute onset, constant, midepigastric or periumbilical abdominal pain radiating to back, often with nausea/vomiting

H/o of gallstones, ETOH abuse, prior pancreatitis, use of medications commonly associated with pancreatitis*

Check serum amylase/lipase — **both normal** → Acute pancreatitis unlikely

either elevated

Are other causes of elevated amylase/lipase ruled out?

yes → **no** → R/O appendicitis, perforated viscus, peptic ulcer, biliary colic, aortic aneurysm, intestinal ischemia, gyn problem, cardiac cause, bowel obstruction

Patient. has pancreatitis (clinical diagnosis)

NPO
IV fluids (pt. usually dehydrated)
Analgesia as needed
NG suction if vomiting

Consider empiric initial therapies of unproven benefit thus far:
- Peritoneal Lavage
- Somatostatin/Octreotide
- Protease inhibitor

Prognosticate via Ranson Criteria† (or APACHE III score)

| ≤ 2 criteria | 3-5 criteria | ≥ 6 criteria |

Mild pancreatitis
<5% morbidity
<1% mortality

Moderate pancreatitis
30% morbidity
5% mortality

Severe pancreatitis
90% morbidity
30% mortality

RUQ ultrasound; bile ducts, GB, liver, pancreas. Evidence for stones?

Aggressive support; ICU

Improvement in first four days?

no → History of previous episode of pancreatitis? **no** / **yes**

yes → • ERCP w/ possible sphincterotomy
• Check bile for microlithiasis,
• Consider cholecystectomy
• Consider sphincter of Oddi manometry.

yes / **no**

CT abdomen with IV contrast. Necrosis present?

no / **yes**

• Await pain resolution
• Supportive care
• OK to eat when pain has resolved

Fevers present?

no / **yes**

• CT guided needle biopsy to r/o infected necrosis
• Empiric antibiotics against enteric pathogens
• Surgical debridement should be strongly considered

*Medications Often Associated with Pancreatitis

Strong Association	Association
Azothioprine	Valproic Acid
6-Mercaptopurine	Sulfonamides
2'-3'-Dideosyinosine	Thiazide diuretics
Pentamidine	Sulfasalazine
	Aminosalicylic acid
	Methyldopa
	Octreotide

†Ranson Criteria

On Admission	Within 48 hrs.
Age >55	Hct drop > 10%
WBC > 16,000/cc	BUN inc. > 5mg/dl
Glucose > 200 mg/dl	Ca < 8 mg/dL
AST > 250 IL/L	pO2 < 60 mm Hg
LDH > 350 IU/L	Base deficit > 4meq/L
	Fluid sequestration > 6L

1. Calleja GA Barkin JS. Acute pancreatitis. Med Clin N Amer 1993 77(5):1037-1056
2. Steinberg W Tenner S Acute pancreatitis NEJM 1994 330 (17):1198-210
3. Marshall JB Acute pancreatitis: a review with an emphasis on new developments. Arch Int Med 1993 153(10):1185-98

5j: Acute Right Upper Quadrant Pain

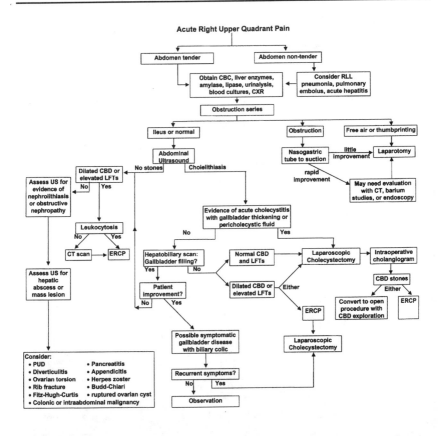

Acute Right Upper Quadrant Pain

Abdomen tender → Obtain CBC, liver enzymes, amylase, lipase, urinalysis, blood cultures, CXR ← Abdomen non-tender → Consider RLL pneumonia, pulmonary embolus, acute hepatitis

Obstruction series

- Ileus or normal → Abdominal Ultrasound
- Obstruction → Nasogastric tube to suction — little improvement → Laparotomy; rapid improvement → May need evaluation with CT, barium studies, or endoscopy
- Free air or thumbprinting → Laparotomy

Abdominal Ultrasound: No stones → Dilated CBD or elevated LFTs (No / Yes); Cholelithiasis

Dilated CBD or elevated LFTs — No → Assess US for evidence of nephrolithiasis or obstructive nephropathy; Yes → Leukocytosis (No → CT scan → ERCP; Yes → ERCP)

Assess US for hepatic abscess or mass lesion

Evidence of acute cholecystitis with gallbladder thickening or pericholecystic fluid: No / Yes

No → Hepatobiliary scan: Gallbladder filling? Yes / No
- Yes → Patient improvement? No / Yes
- No → Normal CBD and LFTs / Dilated CBD or elevated LFTs

Yes → Laparoscopic Cholecystectomy → Intraoperative cholangiogram → CBD stones → Either → Convert to open procedure with CBD exploration / ERCP

Normal CBD and LFTs → Laparoscopic Cholecystectomy
Dilated CBD or elevated LFTs — Either → ERCP

Patient improvement? Yes → Possible symptomatic gallbladder disease with biliary colic → Recurrent symptoms? No → Observation; Yes → Laparoscopic Cholecystectomy

Consider:
- PUD
- Diverticulitis
- Ovarian torsion
- Rib fracture
- Fitz-Hugh-Curtis
- Colonic or intraabdominal malignancy
- Pancreatitis
- Appendicitis
- Herpes zoster
- Budd-Chiari
- ruptured ovarian cyst

Abbreviations: US = ultrasound, CT = computed tomography, ERCP = endoscopic retrograde cholangiopancreatography, CBD = common bile duct, LFTs = liver function tests, PUD = peptic ulcer disease.

Erikson, RA and Carlson, B. The role of endoscopic retrograde cholangiopancreatography in patients with laparoscopic cholecystectomies. Gastroenterology 1995;109:252.

Rathgaber S. Right upper quadrant abdominal pain: Diagnosis in patients without evident gallstones. Postgraduate Med 1993;94:153

Paterson-Brown S, Vipond MN. Modern aids to clinical decision making in the acute abdomen. Br. J. Surg. 1990;77:13.

Brewer RJ, Golden GR, Hitch DC, et al. Abdominal pain: An analysis of 1000 consecutive cases in a university hospital emergency room. Am. J. Surg. 1976;131:219.

Bender JS. Approach to the acute abdomen. Med. Clin. N.A. 1989; 73:1413.

5k: Treatment of Inflammatory Bowel Disease - Crohn's Disease

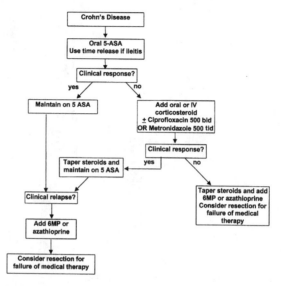

Agents used in the treatment of Inflammatory Bowel Disease

Category	Drug	Unit	Dose range	Site of Release
Oral 5-ASA	Sulfasalazine (Azulfidine)	500 mg	2-4 g/day	colon
Oral 5-ASA	Mesalamine (Asacol)	400 mg	2.4-4.8 g/day	colon/ileum
Oral 5-ASA	Mesalamine time release (Pentasa)	250 mg	3.0-4 g/day	duodenum to colon
Oral 5-ASA	Olsalazine (Dipentum)	250 mg	0.75 - 3.0 g/day	colon/ileum
5-ASA suppository	Mesalamine suppository	0.5 or 1 g	One suppository bid	rectum
5-ASA enema	Mesalamine enema	60 or 100 ml	4 g QD or bid	left colon
Oral corticosteroid	Oral steroid: prednisone*	5-20 mg	40-60 mg/day with subsequent taper	
IV corticosteroid	IV steroid: Hydrocortisone		100 mg Q 8H	
Corticosteroid enema	Hydrocortisone enema*	100 mg	100 mg QD or bid	left colon
Immunosuppressive	6 mercaptopurine	50 mg	1.0 - 1.5 mg/kg/day	
Immunosuppressive	Azathioprine (Imuran)	50 mg	1.0-2.0 mg/kg/day	
Immunosuppressive	IV cyclosporin		4 mg/kg/day	

*Alternate day oral steroids have been shown to reduce side effects. Budesonide may have equal or greater efficacy with less systemic absorption (studies ongoing)
Immunosuppressive agents should be given only by physicians knowledgeable in their use (recommend subspecialist consultation)

5I: Treatment of Inflammatory Bowel Disease - Ulcerative Colitis

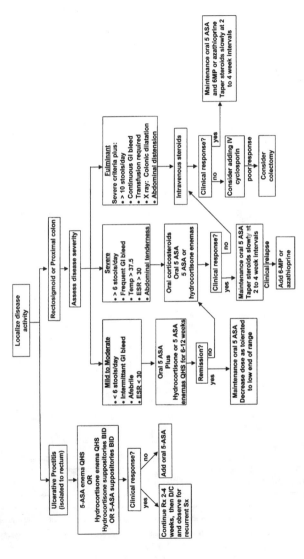

See *Agents used in the treatment of Inflammatory bowel disease* in Crohn's disease algorithm

Elson CO. The basis of current and future therapy for inflammatory bowel disease. Am J Med 100:656- 662, 1996

Pearson DC, May GR, Fick GH, Sutherland LR. Azathioprine and 6 mercaptopurine in Crohn's disease, a meta-analysis. Ann Int Med 123:132-142, 1995

Hanauer SB. Inflammatory Bowel Disease. N Engl J Med 334:841-848, 1996

Sagar PM, Pemberton JH. Update on the surgical management of ulcerative colitis and ulcerative proctitis: current controversies and problems. Inflammatory Bowel Dis 1:299-312, 1996

5m: Elevated Liver Enzymes

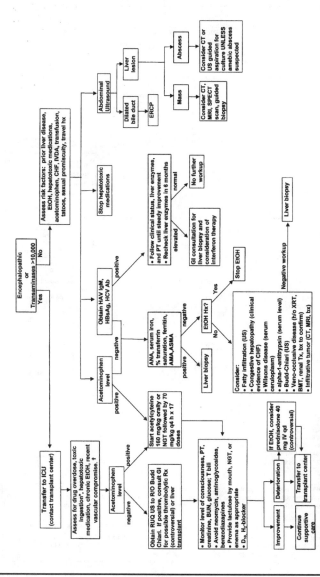

* amanita phalloides, carbon tetrachloride
† Although viral antigens, viral antibodies, and ceruloplasmin should be obtained, they are not helpful in the acute setting. Liver biopsy in general is also not helpful in fulminant hepatic failure.

Abbreviations: EtOH = alcohol, CHF = congestive heart failure, IVDA = intravenous drug abuse, NGT = nasogastric tube, PT = prothrombin time, T Bili = total bilirubin, BUN = blood urea nitrogen, HAV = hepatitis A virus, HBsAg = hepatitis B virus surface antigen, HCV Ab = hepatitis C virus antibody, ANA = antinuclear antibody, AMA = antimitochondrial antibody, ASMA = anti-smooth muscle antibody, ERCP = endoscopic retrograde cholangiopancreatography, CT = computed tomography, MRI = magnetic resonance imaging, US = RUQ ultrasound, D_{10} = 10% dextrose solution.

Herlong HF. Approach to the patient with abnormal liver enzymes. Hospital Practice 1994;29:32.
Lee, WM. Acute liver failure. NEJM 1993;329:1862.
Imperiale, TF, McCullough AJ. Do corticosteroids reduce mortality from alcoholic hepatitis. Ann. Int. Med. 1990;13:299.
Gitlin, NM. Therapeutic implications of the evaluation of liver enzymes. In:Current therapy in gastroenterology and liver disease (ed: T.M. Bayless) Mosby 1994 pg 474.

5n: Upper Gastrointestinal Bleeding

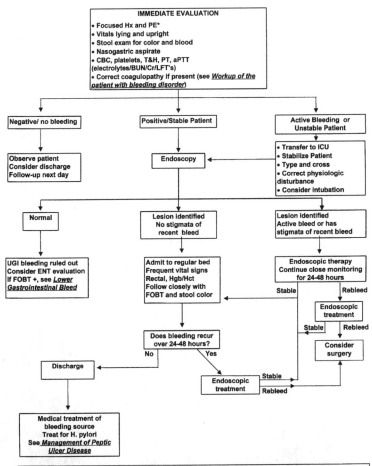

IMMEDIATE EVALUATION
- Focused Hx and PE*
- Vitals lying and upright
- Stool exam for color and blood
- Nasogastric aspirate
- CBC, platelets, T&H, PT, aPTT (electrolytes/BUN/Cr/LFT's)
- Correct coaguolopathy if present (see *Workup of the patient with bleeding disorder*)

Negative/ no bleeding

Observe patient
Consider discharge
Follow-up next day

Positive/Stable Patient

Endoscopy

Active Bleeding or Unstable Patient
- Transfer to ICU
- Stabilize Patient
- Type and cross
- Correct physiologic disturbance
- Consider intubation

Normal

UGI bleeding ruled out
Consider ENT evaluation
If FOBT +, see *Lower Gastrointestinal Bleed*

Lesion identified No stigmata of recent bleed

Admit to regular bed
Frequent vital signs
Rectal, Hgb/Hct
Follow closely with FOBT and stool color

Lesion identified Active bleed or has stigmata of recent bleed

Endoscopic therapy
Continue close monitoring for 24-48 hours

Stable | Rebleed

Endoscopic treatment

Stable | Rebleed

Consider surgery

Does bleeding recur over 24-48 hours?
No | Yes

Discharge

Endoscopic treatment
Stable | Rebleed

Medical treatment of bleeding source
Treat for H. pylori
See *Management of Peptic Ulcer Disease*

*Focused H&P vitals: Prompt initial exam should determine severity of situation. Evaluation of vitals, particularly for orthostatic changes , is critical. History should determine likely cause of bleeding (liver disease, NSAIDS, vomiting, ulcer, cancer, etc.) All patients need rectal exam and naso-gastric lavage.

Immediate Laboratory Evaluation: Includes CBC (with platelets, MCV) protime, electrolytes, BUN/Cr, and type and hold or cross. Consider obtaining LFT's, bleeding time, alcohol level, toxicology screen as appropriate.

Risk Factors: Morbidity, mortality and risk for rebleeding increase with these risk factors: rebleeding, large volume bleed, bleeding while on treatment, recent ASA/NSAIDe, liver disease, CHF, CAD, renal failure, respiratory failure, and hematologic malignancy or renal failure.

5o: Lower Gastrointestinal Bleed

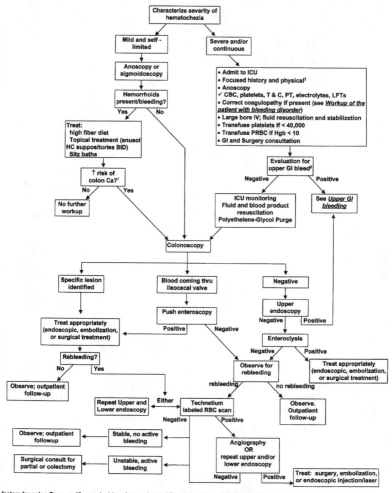

1. Risk factors for colon Ca: age>45, anemia, h/o polyps, colorectal Ca, adenomatous polyps, inflammatory bowel disease, FH of colorectal Ca
2. Signs of upper GI source: Hx of ulcer, liver disease, NSAID use; pain above umbilicus, BUN:Cr>25:1, hyperactive bowels sounds, vomiting, positive nasogastric aspirate

6a: Acute Renal Failure

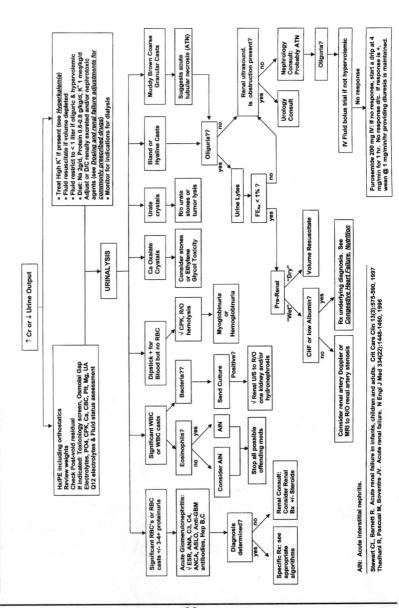

↑ Cr or ↓ Urine Output

Hx/PE including orthostatics
Review weights
Check Post-void residual
If indicated: Toxicology screen, Osmolal Gap
Electrolytes, PO4, CPK, Ca, CBC, Plt, Mg, UA
Q12 electrolytes & Fluid status assessment

- Treat High K⁺ if present (see *Hyperkalemia*)
- Fluid resuscitate if volume depleted
- Fluid restrict to < 1 liter if oliguric & hypervolemic
- Diet: Na 2g/d, Protein 0.6-0.8 g/kg/d, K⁺ 1 meq/kg/d
  Adjust or D/C renally excreted and/or nephrotoxic
  agents (see *Dosing and renal failure adjustments for
  commonly prescribed drugs*)
- Monitor for indications for dialysis

URINALYSIS

Muddy Brown Coarse Granular Casts → Suggests acute tubular necrosis (ATN)

Bland or Hyaline Casts

Urate crystals → R/o urate stones or tumor lysis

Ca Oxalate Crystals → Consider stones or Ethylene Glycol Toxicity

Dipstick + for Blood but no RBC → √ CPK, R/O hemolysis → Myoglobinuria or Hemoglobinuria

Significant WBC or WBC casts

Bacteria?? → Send Culture → Positive? → √ Renal U/S to R/O one kidney and/or hydronephrosis

Eosinophils? → yes → AIN
no → Consider AIN → Stop all possible offending meds

Significant RBC's or RBC casts +/- 3-4+ proteinuria

Acute Glomerulonephritis:
√ ESR, ANA, C3, C4,
ANCA, ASLO, Anti-GBM
antibodies, Hep B,C

Diagnosis determined? → yes → Specific Rx: see appropriate algorithms
no → Renal Consult: Consider Renal Bx +/- Steroids

Oliguria?? → yes → Urine Lytes → FE_Na < 1% ? → yes → Pre-Renal → "Dry" → Volume Resuscitate
"Wet" → CHF or low Albumin? → yes → Rx underlying diagnosis. See *Congestive Heart Failure, Nutrition*
no → Consider renal artery Doppler or MRI to R/O renal artery stenosis

no → Renal ultrasound. Is obstruction present? → yes → Urology Consult
no → Nephrology Consult: Probably ATN → Oliguria?

IV Fluid bolus trial if not hypervolemic
No response

Furosemide 200 mg IV: If no response, start a drip at 4
mg/min for 1 hr. No response d/c. If response is +,
wean @ 1 mg/min/hr providing diuresis is maintained.

AIN: Acute interstitial nephritis.

Stewart CL, Barnett R. Acute renal failure in infants, children and adults. Crit Care Clin 13(3):575-590, 1997
Thadhani R, Pascual M, Boventre JV. Acute renal failure. N Engl J Med 334(22):1448-1460, 1996

6b: Hypertension - Outpatient Therapy

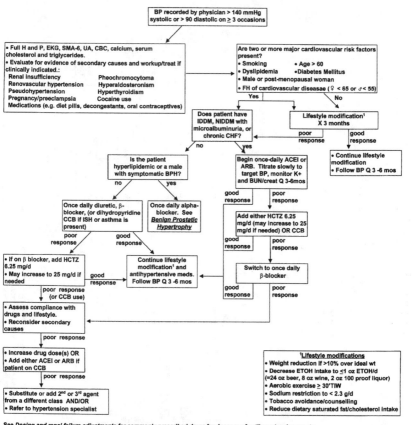

BP recorded by physician > 140 mmHg systolic or > 90 diastolic on ≥ 3 occasions

- Full H and P, EKG, SMA-6, UA, CBC, calcium, serum cholesterol and triglycerides.
- Evaluate for evidence of secondary causes and workup/treat if clinically indicated.:

Renal insufficiency	Pheochromocytoma
Renovascular hypertension	Hyperaldosteronism
Pseudohypertension	Hyperthyroidism
Pregnancy/preeclampsia	Cocaine use

Medications (e.g. diet pills, decongestants, oral contraceptives)

Are two or more major cardiovascular risk factors present?
- Smoking
- Age > 60
- Dyslipidemia
- Diabetes Mellitus
- Male or post-menopausal woman
- FH of cardiovascular diseasae (♀ < 65 or ♂ < 55)

Yes → Does patient have IDDM, NIDDM with microalbuminuria, or chronic CHF?

No → Lifestyle modification[1] X 3 months
- poor response
- good response → • Continue lifestyle modification • Follow BP Q 3 -6 mos

Does patient have IDDM, NIDDM with microalbuminuria, or chronic CHF?
- **no** → Is the patient hyperlipidemic or a male with symptomatic BPH?
- **yes** → Begin once-daily ACEI or ARB. Titrate slowly to target BP, monitor K+ and BUN/creat Q 3-6mos

Is the patient hyperlipidemic or a male with symptomatic BPH?
- **no** → Once daily diuretic, β-blocker, (or dihydropyridine CCB if ISH or asthma is present)
- **yes** → Once daily alpha-blocker. See ***Benign Prostatic Hypertrophy***

Once daily diuretic, β-blocker, (or dihydropyridine CCB if ISH or asthma is present)
- poor response → • If on β blocker, add HCTZ 6.25 mg/d • May increase to 25 mg/d if needed
- good response → Continue lifestyle modification[1] and antihypertensive meds. Follow BP Q 3 -6 mos

Begin once-daily ACEI or ARB. Titrate slowly to target BP, monitor K+ and BUN/creat Q 3-6mos
- good response
- poor response → Add either HCTZ 6.25 mg/d (may increase to 25 mg/d if needed) OR CCB
  - good response
  - poor response → Switch to once daily β-blocker
    - good response
    - poor response → (continues)

• If on β blocker, add HCTZ 6.25 mg/d
• May increase to 25 mg/d if needed
- good response → Continue lifestyle modification[1] and antihypertensive meds. Follow BP Q 3 -6 mos
- poor response (or CCB use) →

• Assess compliance with drugs and lifestyle.
• Reconsider secondary causes
- poor response →

• Increase drug dose(s) OR
• Add either ACEI or ARB if patient on CCB
- poor response →

• Substitute or add 2nd or 3rd agent from a different class AND/OR
• Refer to hypertension specialist

[1]Lifestyle modifications
- Weight reduction if >10% over ideal wt
- Decrease ETOH intake to ≤1 oz ETOH/d (=24 oz beer, 8 oz wine, 2 oz 100 proof liquor)
- Aerobic exercise ≥ 30'TIW
- Sodium restriction to < 2.3 g/d
- Tobacco avoidance/counselling
- Reduce dietary saturated fat/cholesterol intake

See *Dosing and renal failure adjustments for commonly prescribed drugs* for dosages of antihypertensive agents.
ACEI - Angiotensin converting enzyme inhibitor. ARB – angiotensin II receptor blocker. ACEIs and ARBs are contraindicated in pregnancy.
Pregnant patients, regardless of coexistent medical conditions, should be trezted with hydralazine or a beta-blocker. African Americans should be offered ACEI but are less likely than Caucasians to respond. A CCB may need to be substituted.
BPH - Benign prostatic hyperplasia. CCB - calcium-channel blockers. ISH - isolated systolic hypertension
HCTZ - hydrochlorthiazide

The Sixth Report of the Joint National Committee on Detection, Evaluation, and Treatment of High Blood Pressure. Arch Int Med 1997; 157:2413-46
Kaplan NM, Lieberman E. Clinical Hypertension. Baltimore, Williams & Wilkins; 180-192, 1990
Alderman MH. Which antihypertensive drugs first -- and why! JAMA 267: 2786 -2787, 1992

6c: Management of Acute Renal Colic

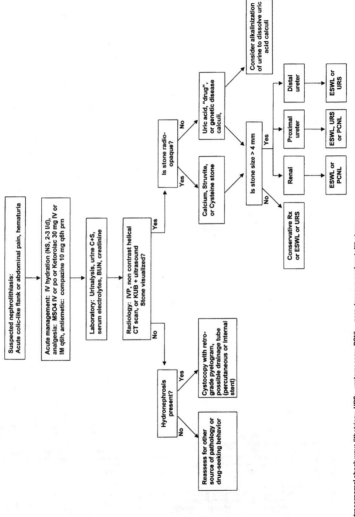

ESWL – extracorporeal shock wave lithotripsy, URS – ureteroscopy, PCNL – percutaneous nephrostolithotomy

Saklayen MG. Medical management of nephrolithiasis. Med Clin NA 81: 785-799, 1997
Segura JW, Preminger GM, Assimos DG et al. Ureteral stones clinical guidelines panel summary report on the management of ureteral calculi. www.auanet.org/guidelines

68

6d: Metabolic Evaluation for Renal Calculi

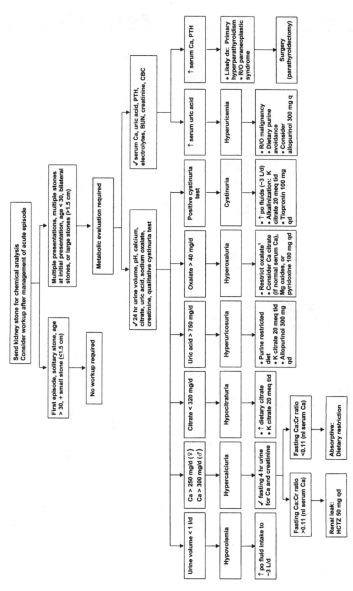

1. Foods which increase urinary oxalate: spinach, rhubarb, chocolate, peanuts, strawberry, tea, wheat bran, ascorbic acid

Saklayen MG. Medical management of nephrolithiasis. Med Clin NA 81: 785-799, 1997
Segura JW, Preminger GM, Assimos DG et al. Ureteral stones clinical guidelines panel summary report on the management of ureteral calculi. www.auanet.org/guidelines

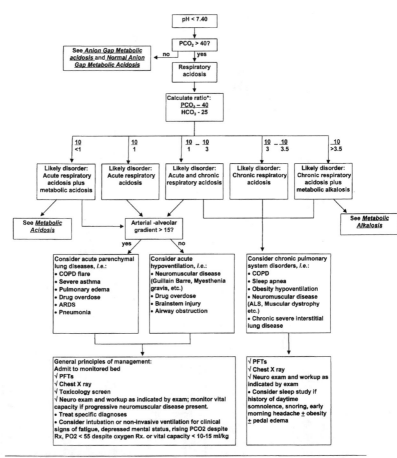

*These ratios can be estimated, but for some you will need a calculator. For a patient with a pCO2 of 45 and bicarb of 32, the ratio would be (45-40)/(32-25) = 5/7 = 10/14. A patient with a pCO2 of 53 with a bicarb of 28 would have a ratio of (53-40)/(28-25) = 13/3 = 10/2.3.

Ratios within these ranges are consistent with, but not necessarily diagnostic of the disorders described. Complex acid-base disorders may mimic simple disorders. History and clinical correlation are required for interpretation.

6f: Anion Gap Metabolic Acidosis

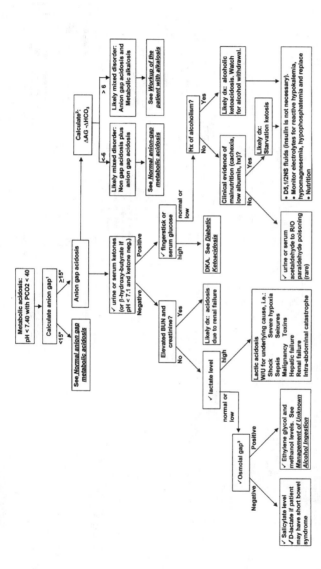

1. Anion gap: Na - (Cl+HCO3). The upper limit of normal will vary with the laboratory, check with your laboratory normals. The anion gap threshold is also lower if the albumin is < 4. If the measured anion gap - [12-2.5(4-albumin)] is > 2, then anion gap acidosis is present.

2. ΔAG = calculated anion gap - 15; ΔHCO₃ = HCO3 - 25. Some authors use ± 8 as cutoff. ΔAG within this range likely have a pure anion gap acidosis, ΔAG outside this range most commonly have the mixed disorders identified above. History and clinical correlation are required for interpretation.

3. Osmolal gap: Measured osmolality – calculated osmolality. Calculated Osm = 2(Na) + Glucose/18 + BUN/2.8 + ethanol/4.6

Wrenn K. The delta gap: An approach to mixed acid base disorders. Ann Emerg Med 19: 1310-1313, 1990
Oster JR, Perez GO, Materson BJ. Use of the anion gap in clinical medicine. So Med J 81:229-237, 1988

71

6g: Normal Anion Gap Metabolic Acidosis

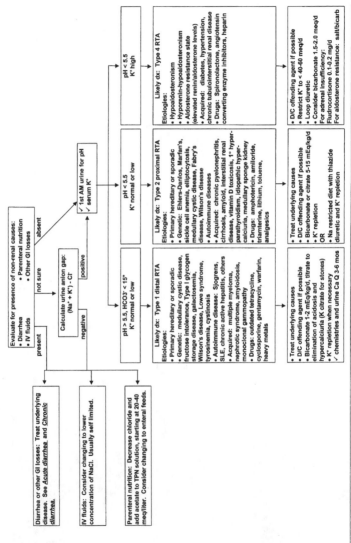

Evaluate for presence of non-renal causes:
- Diarrhea
- IV fluids
- Parenteral nutrition
- Other GI losses

present / **not sure** / **absent**

Calculate urine anion gap:
(Na⁺ + K⁺) - Cl⁻

negative / **positive**

✓ 1st AM urine for pH
✓ serum K⁺

pH > 5.5, HCO3⁻ < 15*
K⁺ normal or low

pH < 5.5
K⁺ normal or low

pH < 5.5
K⁺ high

Diarrhea or other GI losses: Treat underlying disease. See *Acute diarrhea* and *Chronic diarrhea*.

IV fluids: Consider changing to lower concentration of NaCl. Usually self limited.

Parenteral nutrition: Decrease chloride and add acetate to TPN solution, starting at 20-40 meq/liter. Consider changing to enteral feeds.

Likely dx: Type 1 distal RTA
Etiologies:
- Primary hereditary or sporadic
- Genetic: medullary cystic disease, fructose intolerance, Type 1 glycogen storage disease, galactosemia, Wilson's disease, Lowe syndrome, tyrosinemia, cystinosis
- Autoimmune disease: Sjogrens, SLE, chronic active hepatitis, others
- Acquired: multiple myeloma, nephrotic syndrome, amyloidosis, monoclonal gammopathy
- Drugs: outdated tetracycline, cyclosporine, gentamycin, warfarin, heavy metals

- Treat underlying causes
- D/C offending agent if possible
- Bicarbonate 1-2 mEq/kg/d, titrate to elimination of acidosis and hypercalciuria (K citrate for stones)
- K⁺ repletion when necessary
- ✓ chemistries and urine Ca Q 3-6 mos

Likely dx: Type 2 proximal RTA
Etiologies:
- Primary hereditary or sporadic
- Genetic: Ehlers-Danlos, Marfan's, sickle cell anemia, elliptocytosis, medullary cystic disease, Fabry's disease, Wilson's disease
- Autoimmune diseases
- Acquired: chronic pyelonephritis, cirrhosis, amyloid, interstitial renal disease, vitamin D toxicosis, 1° hyperparathyroidism, idiopathic hypercalciuria, medullary sponge kidney
- Drugs: amphotericin, amiloride, triamterene, lithium, toluene, analgesics

- Treat underlying causes
- D/C offending agent if possible
- Bicarbonate or citrate 5-15 mEq/kg/d
- K⁺ repletion
  OR
- Na restricted diet with thiazide diuretic and K⁺ repletion

Likely dx: Type 4 RTA
Etiologies:
- Hypoaldosteronism
- Hyporenin-hypoaldosteronism
- Aldosterone resistance state (elevated renin/aldosterone levels)
- Acquired: diabetes, hypertension, chronic tubulointerstitial renal disease
- Drugs: Spironolactone, angiotensin converting enzyme inhibitors, heparin

- D/C offending agent if possible
- Restrict K⁺ to < 40-60 meq/d
- Loop diuretic
- Consider bicarbonate 1.5-2.0 meq/d
- For adrenal insufficiency:
  Fludrocortisone 0.1-0.2 mg/d
- For aldosterone resistance: salt/bicarb

* If serum bicarbonate > 15, may be type I or type II. Consult renal for urine acidification tests.

Smulders YM et al. Renal tubular acidosis: pathophysiology and diagnosis. Arch Intern Med 156: 1629-1636, 1996

Battle et al. The use of the urinary anion gap in the diagnosis of hyperchloremic metabolic acidosis. N Engl J Med 318: 594-599, 1988

Coe FL, Kathpalia S. Hereditary tubular disorders. in Isselbacher KJ, et al, eds., Harrison's Principles of Internal Medicine, 13th ed., McGraw Hill, New York, 1326-1329, 1994

6h: Workup of the Patient with Alkalosis

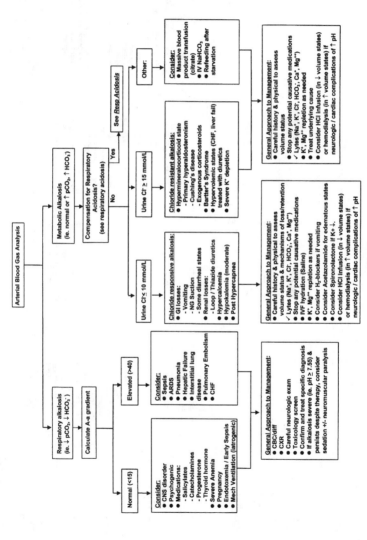

Arterial Blood Gas Analysis

Respiratory alkalosis (ie. ↓ pCO₂, ↓ HCO₃⁻)

Calculate A-a gradient

Normal (<15)
Consider:
- CNS disorder
- Psychogenic
- Medications:
  - Salicylates
  - Catecholamines
  - Progesterone
  - Thyroid hormone
- Severe Anemia
- Pregnancy
- Endotoxemia / Early Sepsis
- Mech Ventilation (iatrogenic)

Elevated (>40)
Consider:
- Sepsis
- ARDS
- Pneumonia
- Hepatic Failure
- Interstitial lung disease
- Pulmonary Embolism
- CHF

General Approach to Management:
- CBC/diff
- CXR
- Careful neurologic exam
- Toxicology screen
- Confirm and treat specific diagnosis
- If alkalosis severe (ie. pH ≥ 7.55) & persists despite therapy, consider sedation +/- neuromuscular paralysis

Metabolic Alkalosis (ie. normal or ↑ pCO₂, ↑ HCO₃⁻)

Compensation for Respiratory Acidosis? (see respiratory acidosis)

Yes → See *Resp Acidosis*

No ↓

Urine Cl⁻ ≤ 10 mmol/L

Chloride responsive alkalosis:
- GI losses:
  - Vomiting
  - NG Suction
  - Some diarrheal states
- Renal losses
  - Loop / Thiazide diuretics
- Hypercalcemia
- Hypokalemia (moderate)
- Post Hypercapnea

General Approach to Management:
- Careful history & physical to assess volume status & mechanisms of loss/retention
- Stop any potential causative medications
- ✓ Lytes (Na⁺, K⁺, Cl⁻, HCO₃⁻, Ca⁺, Mg⁺⁺)
- IVF hydration (Saline)
- K⁺, Mg⁺⁺ repletion as needed
- Consider H₂-blockers if vomiting
- Consider Acetazolamide for edematous states
- Consider Spironolactone if ↑ K+↓
- Consider HCl Infusion (in ↓ volume states) or hemodialysis (in ↑ volume states) if neurologic / cardiac complications of ↑ pH

Urine Cl⁻ ≥ 15 mmol/L

Chloride resistant alkalosis:
- Hypermineralocorticoid state
  - Primary hyperaldosteronism
  - Cushing's disease
  - Exogenous corticosteroids
- Bartter's Syndrome
- Hypovolemic states (CHF, liver fail) treated with diuretics
- Severe K⁺ depletion

Other:
Consider:
- Massive blood product transfusion (citrate)
- IV NaHCO₃
- Refeeding after starvation

General Approach to Management:
- Careful history & physical to assess volume status
- Stop any potential causative medications
- ✓ Lytes (Na⁺, K⁺, Cl⁻, HCO₃⁻, Ca⁺, Mg⁺⁺)
- K⁺, Mg⁺⁺ repletion as needed
- Treat underlying cause
- Consider HCl Infusion (in ↓ volume states) or hemodialysis (in ↑ volume states) if neurologic / cardiac complications of ↑ pH

1. Black, RM. Metabolic Acidosis and Metabolic Alkalosis. In *Intensive Care Medicine*: Rippe, Irwin, Fink, Cerra (eds) 3ʳᵈ ed. Little Brown & Co. Boston, 1996. Chapter 80, pp 993 - 998.
2. Don, H Metabolic Alkalosis. In *Decision Making in Critical Care*: Don (ed.) BC Decker, Inc. Philadelphia, 1985. Pages 166 - 167.

7a: Treatment of Anaphylactic and Anaphylactoid Reactions

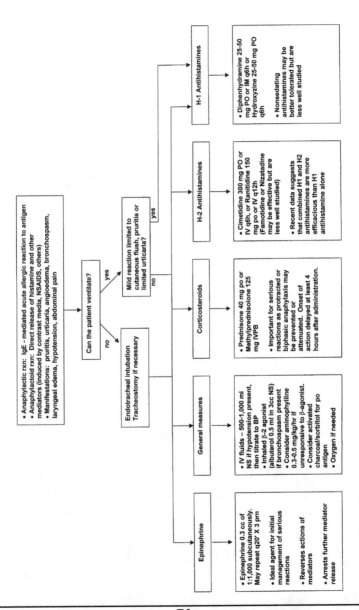

- Anaphylactic rxn: IgE - mediated acute allergic reaction to antigen
- Anaphylactoid rxn: Direct release of histamine and other mediators (induced by contrast media, NSAIDS, others)
- Manifestations: pruritis, urticaria, angioedema, bronchospasm, laryngeal edema, hypotension, abdominal pain

Can the patient ventilate?

→ no → Endotracheal intubation / Tracheostomy if necessary

→ yes → **Mild reaction limited to cutaneous flush, pruritis or limited urticaria?**

→ no → (to General measures / Corticosteroids / H-2 Antihistamines)

→ yes → (to H-1 Antihistamines)

Epinephrine
- Epinephrine 0.3 cc of 1:1,000 subcutaneously. May repeat q20" X 3 prn
- Ideal agent for initial management of serious reactions
- Reverses actions of mediators
- Arrests further mediator release

General measures
- IV fluids – 500-1,000 ml NS if hypotension present, then titrate to BP
- Inhaled β-2 agonist (albuterol 0.5 ml in 3cc NS) if bronchospasm present
- Consider aminophylline 0.3-0.5 mg/kg/hr if unresponsive to β-agonist.
- Consider activated charcoal/sorbitol for po antigen
- Oxygen if needed

Corticosteroids
- Prednisone 40 mg po or Methylprednisolone 125 mg IVPB
- Important for serious reactions as protracted or biphasic anaphylaxis may be prevented or attenuated. Onset of action delayed at least 4 hours after administration.

H-2 Antihistamines
- Cimetidine 300 mg PO or IV q6h, or Ranitidine 150 mg po or IV q12h (Famotidine or Nizatadine may be effective but are less well studied)
- Recent data suggests that combined H1 and H2 antihistamines are more efficacious than H1 antihistamine alone

H-1 Antihistamines
- Diphenhydramine 25-50 mg PO or IM q6h or Hydroxyzine 25-50 mg PO q8h
- Nonsedating antihistamines may be better tolerated but are less well studied

Bochner BS, Lichtenstein LM. Anaphylaxis. N Engl J Med 324: 1785-1790, 1991
Stark BJ, Sullivan TJ. Biphasic and protracted anaphylaxis. J Allergy Clin Immunol 78: 76-83, 1986
Lang DM. Anaphylactoid and anaphylactic reactions: Hazards of β-adrenergic blockers. Drug Safety 12: 299-304, 1995

7b: Insect Stings: Management and Prevention of Anaphylactic Reactions from Hymenoptera Venom

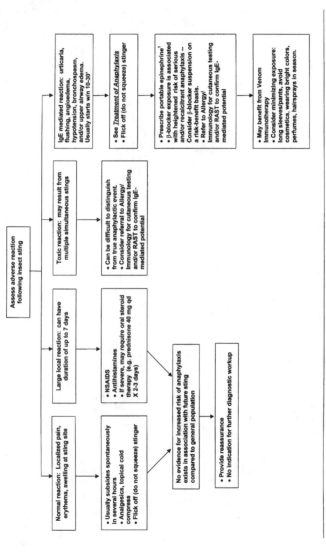

```
                    Assess adverse reaction
                     following insect sting
```

Normal reaction: Localized pain, erythema, swelling at sting site
- Usually subsides spontaneously in several hours
- Analgesics, topical cold compress
- Flick off (do not squeeze) stinger

Large local reaction: can have duration of up to 7 days
- NSAIDS
- Antihistamines
- If severe, may require oral steroid therapy (e.g. prednisone 40 mg qd X 2-3 days)

No evidence for increased risk of anaphylaxis exists in association with future sting compared to general population
- Provide reassurance
- No indication for further diagnostic workup

Toxic reaction: may result from multiple simultaneous stings
- Can be difficult to distinguish from true anaphylactic event.
- Consider referral to Allergy/ Immunology for cutaneous testing and/or RAST to confirm IgE-mediated potential

IgE mediated reaction: urticaria, flushing, angioedema, hypotension, bronchospasm, and/or upper airway edema. Usually starts w/n 10-30'
- See *Treatment of Anaphylaxis*
- Flick off (do not squeeze) stinger

- Prescribe portable epinephrine[1]
- β-blocker exposure is associated with heightened risk of serious and/or recalcitrant anaphylaxis – Consider β-blocker suspension on a risk-benefit basis.
- Refer to Allergy/ Immunology for cutaneous testing and/or RAST to confirm IgE-mediated potential

- May benefit from Venom Immunotherapy
- Consider minimizing exposure: long sleeves/pants, avoid cosmetics, wearing bright colors, perfumes, hairsprays in season.

Portable epinephrine: 0.3 ml of 1:1,000 epinephrine (EpiPen, ANA-kit, ANA-guard – also contains 2 mg tablets of chlorpheniramine maleate)
Hymenoptera: Honeybees, Vespids (yellow jacket, hornet), wasp

Golden DBK, Marsh DG, Kagey-Sobotka A, Friedhoff L, Szklo M, Valentine MD, Lichtenstein LM. Epidemiology of insect venom sensitivity. JAMA 262: 240-244, 1989
Valentine MD. Allergy to stinging insects. Ann Allergy 70: 427-432, 1993
Levine MI, Lockey RF. Monograph on Insect Allergy (3rd Edition). American Acadamy of Allergy and Immunology, Dave Lambert Associates, Pittsburgh, PA, 1995.

7c: Prevention of Anaphylactoid Reactions From Contrast Media

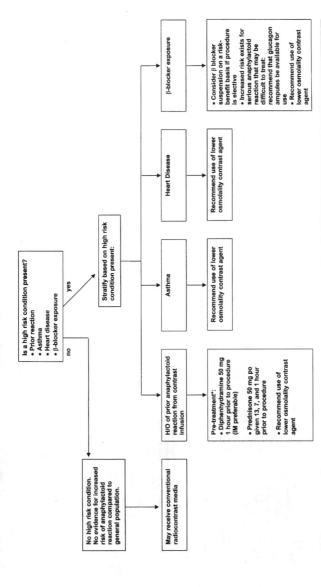

Is a high risk condition present?
- Prior reaction
- Asthma
- Heart disease
- β-blocker exposure

no → **No high risk condition. No evidence for increased risk of anaphylactoid reaction compared to general population.** → **May receive conventional radiocontrast media**

yes → **Stratify based on high risk condition present:**

H/O of prior anaphylactoid reaction from contrast infusion

Pre-treatment*:
- Diphenhydramine 50 mg 1 hour prior to procedure (IM preferable)
- Prednisone 50 mg po given 13, 7, and 1 hour prior to procedure
- Recommend use of lower osmolality contrast agent

Asthma

Recommend use of lower osmolality contrast agent

Heart Disease

Recommend use of lower osmolality contrast agent

β-blocker exposure

- Consider β blocker suspension on a risk-benefit basis if procedure is elective
- Increased risk exists for serious anaphylactoid reaction that may be difficult to treat: recommend that glucagon ampules be available for use
- Recommend use of lower osmolality contrast agent

Greenberger PA, Patterson R, Tapio CM. Prophylaxis against repeated radiocontrast media reactions in 857 cases. Arch Intern Med 145: 2197-2200, 1985
Jacobson PD, Rosenquist J. The introduction of low-osmolar contrast agents in radiology: medical, economic, legal and public policy issues. JAMA 268: 1568-1592, 1988
Katayama H, Yagamuchi K, et al. Adverse reactions to ionic and nonionic contrast media. Radiology 175: 621-626, 1990
Lang DM, Alpern MB, Visintainer PF, Smith ST. Elevated risk for anaphylactoid reaction from radiographic contrast media is associated with both β-adrenergic blocker exposure and cardiovascular disorders. Arch Intern Med 153: 2033-2040, 1993
Lang DM. Anaphylactoid and anaphylactic reactions: Hazards of β blockers. Drug Safety 12: 299-304, 1995
Lieberman P. Anaphylactoid reactions to radiocontrast material. Immunol Allergy Clin NA 12: 649-670, 1992
Manual on Iodinated Contrast Material. American College of Radiology, 1990
* Pretreatment with/without use of low osmolar contrast agent reduces (but does not eliminate) risk for anaphylactoid reaction.

7d: Management of Patients with Penicillin Allergy

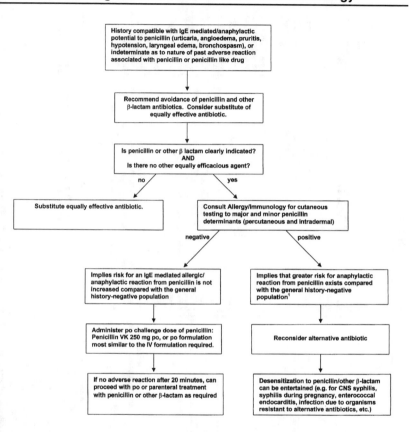

History compatible with IgE mediated/anaphylactic potential to penicillin (urticaria, angioedema, pruritis, hypotension, laryngeal edema, bronchospasm), or indeterminate as to nature of past adverse reaction associated with penicillin or penicillin like drug

Recommend avoidance of penicillin and other β-lactam antibiotics. Consider substitute of equally effective antibiotic.

Is penicillin or other β lactam clearly indicated?
AND
Is there no other equally efficacious agent?

no / yes

Substitute equally effective antibiotic.

Consult Allergy/Immunology for cutaneous testing to major and minor penicillin determinants (percutaneous and intradermal)

negative / positive

Implies risk for an IgE mediated allergic/anaphylactic reaction from penicillin is not increased compared with the general history-negative population

Implies that greater risk for anaphylactic reaction from penicillin exists compared with the general history-negative population[1]

Administer po challenge dose of penicillin: Penicillin VK 250 mg po, or po formulation most similar to the IV formulation required.

Reconsider alternative antibiotic

If no adverse reaction after 20 minutes, can proceed with po or parenteral treatment with penicillin or other β-lactam as required

Desensitization to penicillin/other β-lactam can be entertained (e.g. for CNS syphilis, syphilis during pregnancy, enterococcal endocarditis, infection due to organisms resistant to alternative antibiotics, etc.)

1. Administration of other β-lactams, including carbopenims and cephalosporins may entail greater risk of anaphylaxis in penicillin allergic patients. For this reason, administration of other β-lactams should be avoided if possible.

Saxon A, Beall GN, Rohr AS, Adelman DC. Immediate hypersensitivity reactions to β-lactam antibiotics. Ann Intern Med 107: 204-215, 1987

Sogn DD, Evans R, Shepherd GM et al. National Institute of Allergy and Infectious Diseases, Bethesda MD and other centers: Results of the National Institute of Allergy and Infectious Diseases collaborative clinical trial to test the predictive value of skin testing with major and minor penicillin derivatives in hospitalized adults. Arch Intern Med 152: 1025-1032, 1992

7e: Nasal Miseries

Diagnosis	Allergic rhinitis (AR)	NARES[1]	Nasal polyps	Vasomotor rhinitis	Chronic Sinusitis	Rhinitis Medicamentosa
Symptoms	Pruritis, congestion, clear discharge, sneezing	Clear discharge; ± pruritis	Congestion, clear discharge, *usually unilateral*	Severe congestion with copious clear discharge	Cough, URI symptoms	Congestion and rhinorrhea
Occurrence	Seasonal or perennial	Perennial	Perennial	Perennial	Perennial	Perennial
Onset	Any age	Adult	Usually adult	Adult	Any age	Any age
Associated Factors	Asthma, allergic conjunctivitis	Asthma, aspirin sensitivity	Asthma, aspirin sensitivity, allergic rhinitis (AR), cystic fibrosis, sinusitis	Women > men, sx increase with enviornmental and physical factors (temperature, ETOH, humidity, stress, strong odor, spicy foods)	Possible structural abnormalities, post viral URI, AR, rarely tumors	History of chronic topical decongestant use, oral antihypertensives, psychotropic drugs, or oral birth control pills
Nasal mucosa	Pale/Blue	Pale/Blue	Pale/blue gelatinous ("bag of jelly")	Edema	Red with edema	Bright red with edema
Nasal smear	Eosinophils	Eosinophils	Eosinophils	Normal	PMNs	Normal
Skin test	Positive	Negative	Negative unless associated with AR	Negative unless associated with AR	Negative unless associated with AR	Negative
Etiology	IgE mediated	Unknown	Unknown – outpouching of lining of sinuses	Possibly autonomic dysfunction	Bacterial infection	Tachyphylaxis to topical decongestants with "rebound" congestion and rhinorrhea
Treatment	Avoidance, oral antihistamines, nasal steroids, nasal ipratropium bromide	Nasal steroids, nasal ipratropium bromide	Nasal steroids, treatment of AR or sinusitis if present, surgery if Rx fails.	Nasal steroids, oral decongestants, nasal ipratropium bromide	Antibiotics[3], nasal or oral decongestants, nasal Ipratropium bromide	Stop offending medication[2]; nasal ± oral steroids, nasal ipratropium bromide

Oral nonsedating antihistamines: Astemizole 10 mg qd, Cetirizine10 mg qd, Fexofenadine 60 mg qd, Loratadine 10 mg qd. 1st generation antihistamines may be equally effective and are less expensive.

Nasal steroids: Beclomethasone 1 puff in each nostril bid-qid, Budesonide 2 sprays in each nostril bid, Mometasone 2 sprays in each nostril qd, Flunisolide 2 sprays in each nostril bid, or Triamcinolone 1-2 sprays in each nostril qd

Ipratropium bromide 0.03%: 2 puffs in each nostril bid-tid for above indications. Ipratropium bromide 0.06%: 2 puffs in each nostril tid - qid X 4 days for common cold.

Oral decongestants: Pseudoephedrine 120 mg sustained release q12h, phenylpropanolamine 75 mg sustained release q12h; many preparations have guiafenesin.

Mucus thinning agent: Guiafenesin 400-1200 mg bid

1. NARES – nonallergic rhinitis with eosinophils syndrome
2. If topical agent, consider withdrawing medication one nostril at a time
3. Antibiotics: Amoxicillin/clavulinic acid 875 mg bid, TMP/SMX 1 DS BID, or cefuroxime axetil 250 mg bid for 3 weeks depending on chronicity

Meltzer EO. Anticholinergic therapy for allergic and nonallergic rhinitis and the common cold. J All Clin Immunol 95(5 pt 2) May 1995
Kaliner M, Lemanske R. Rhinitis and Asthma, in Primer on Allergic and Immunologic Disease. JAMA 268: 2807-2829, 1992

7f: Diagnostic Workup of Recurrent Infections

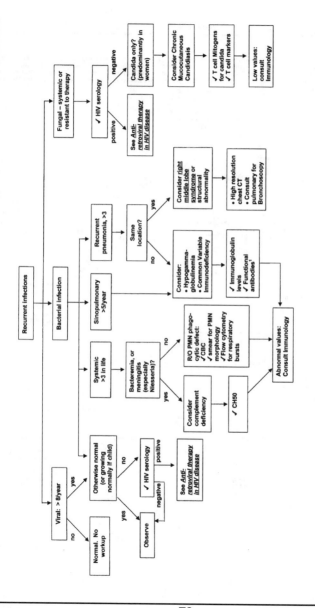

Stiehm ER. New and old immunodeficiencies. Pediatr Res (33 suppl): S2-S8, 1993
Johnson RB Jr. Recurrent bacterial infections in children. N Engl J Med 310:237-243, 1984

1. Antibodies vs. tetanus, pneumococcus, and/or H influenza. If negative, confirm by giving Pneumovacs vaccine and look for response. Lack of response is c/w B-cell defect and Immunology should be consulted.

8a: Anemia

The etiology of most anemias in adults is easily definable with a careful history, physical, and a minimum of diagnostic studies. However, these studies must be obtained prior to transfusion or initiation of therapy. There are in essence, only two causes of anemia: failure of production and increased destruction. Two readily obtainable pieces of information are all that are required to determine further work-up: (1) Classification of anemia: MCV and (2) Evaluation of marrow response: reticulocyte index (RI). RI = % reticulocytes X patient Hct/normal Hct. Divide RI by 2 if nucleated RBCs are present.

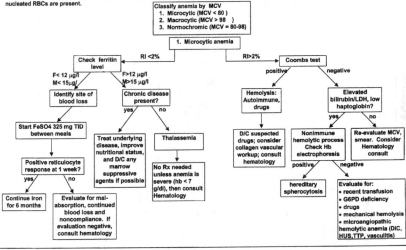

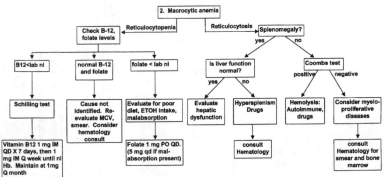

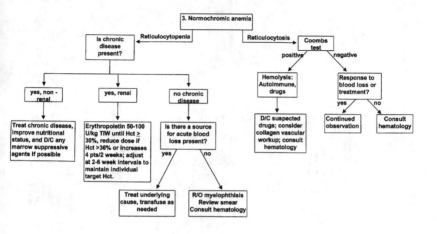

Summary

The common causes of microcytic anemia:
- Iron deficiency
- Thalassemia
- Chronic disease

The common causes of macrocytic anemia:
- B-12 and folate deficiency
- Liver disease
- Reticulocytosis

The common causes of normochromic anemia:
- Chronic disease
- Early acute blood loss
- Intrinsic defects

8b: Workup of the Patient with Bleeding Disorder

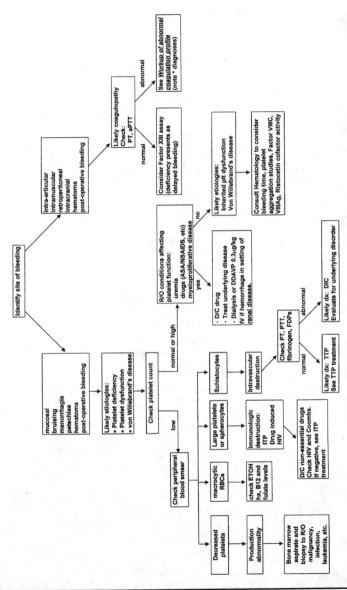

Coller BS and Schneiderman PI. Clinical evaluation of hemorrhagic disorders: Bleeding history and differential diagnosis of purpura. In Hoffman R, Benz EJ, Shattil SJ, Furie B, Cohen HJ, and Silberstein LE eds., Hematology, Basic Principles and Practice, Churchill Livingstone, New York 1995 p. 1606-1622.

8c: Workup of the Patient with Hypercoagulable State

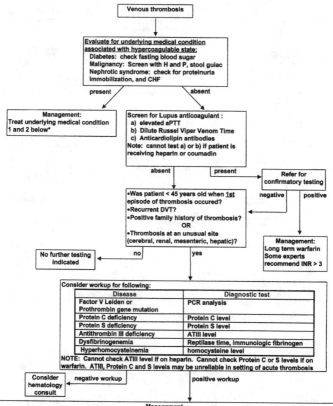

Note: Pregnant women with thrombosis should be treated with heparin. They should not receive warfarin.

1. Schulman S, Grandqvist S, Holmstrom M, et al. The duration of oral anticoagulation therapy after a second episode of venous thromboembolism. N Engl J Med 336: 393-8, 1997

2. DeStefano V, Finazzi G, Mannucci PM. Inherited Thrombophilia: pathogenesis, clinical syndromes, and management. Blood 87: 3531-3544, 1996

3. Bauer KA. Management of patients with hereditary defects predisposing to thrombosis including pregnant women. Thrombosis and Haemostasis 74:94-100, 1995

8d: Workup of Abnormal Coagulation Profile

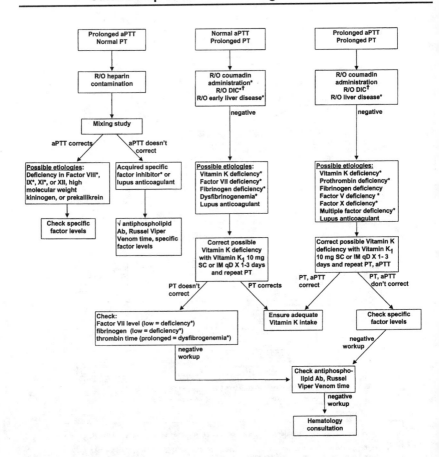

*Associated with bleeding disorders
† √ platelet count, fibrinogen, fibrin degradation products

Santoro SA and Eby CS. Laboratory evaluation of hemostatic disorders. In Hoffman R, Benz EJ, Shattil SJ, Furie B, Cohen HJ, and Silberstein LE eds., Hematology, Basic Principles and Practice, Churchill Livingstone, New York 1995 p. 1622-1632

8e: Treatment of Bleeding Disorders

Thrombocytopenia: Production abnormality (hematology consult recommended)
Patient not actively bleeding: Transfuse platelets only if less than 10,000 (some recommend 20,000)
Patient actively bleeding: Transfuse if platelet count is less than 50,000

Thrombocytopenia: Destruction abnormality (hematology consult recommended)
TTP: Plasmapheresis
ITP: Steroids: prednisone 1mg/kg/day; taper when plt > 100,000
        IV Gamma Globulin: 0.4 g/kg/day X 5 days or 1 g/kg/day X 2 days
        Splenectomy: if unresponsive to glucocorticoids (give pneumococcal, meningococcal, and H influenza vaccinations prior to splenectomy)

Vitamin K deficiency:
Vitamin K_1 10 mg QD X 1-3 days IM or SC. Patients at risk (e.g. on TPN), should receive prophylactic treatment with vitamin K_1 10 mg po or SC TIW.
Fresh Frozen Plasma: 2-4 units IV if patient is bleeding

Warfarin overdose
Hold warfarin
Low dose Vitamin K_1, 1 mg po or SC, if patient needs to remain therapeutic on warfarin
Vitamin K_1 10 mg IM or SC if hemorrhage present or full correction desired
Fresh Frozen Plasma: 2-4 units IV if hemorrhage present

von Willebrand's Disease
Desmopressin acetate: 0.3 µg/kg IV. May be repeated Q 24H; tachyphylaxis may occur
Virally inactivated von Willebrand Factor concentrate
Cryoprecipitate: 10 bags (if life or limb threatening emergency and virally inactivated concentrate is not available)
Consult Hematology

Factor deficiencies

Multiple factor deficiency:	fresh frozen plasma
Fibrinogen deficiency:	Cryoprecipitate
Factor VIII deficiency:	virus inactivated Factor VIII concentrate, 50u/kg load for 100% replacement
Factor IX deficiency	virus inactivated Factor IX concentrate, 80-100 u/kg load for 100% replacement
Factor XI deficiency:	fresh frozen plasma (Factor XI concentrate NA in USA)

8f: Management of Nonemergent Transfusion Reactions

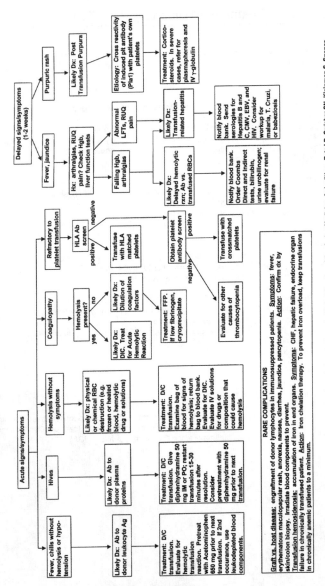

RARE COMPLICATIONS

<u>Graft vs. host disease:</u> engraftment of donor lymphocytes in immunosuppressed patients. In clinical Practice of Transfusion reactions. <u>Symptoms:</u> fever, erythematous maculopapular rash, anorexia, nausea, diarrhea, jaundice, pancytopenia. <u>Action:</u> Confirm dx by skin/colon biopsy. Irradiate blood components to prevent.

<u>Transfusion hemosiderosis:</u> accumulation of iron in end organs. <u>Symptoms:</u> CHF, hepatic failure, endocrine organ failure in chronically transfused patient. <u>Action:</u> Iron chelation therapy. To prevent iron overload, keep transfusions in chronically anemic patients to a minimum.

Jenner PW and Holland PV. The diagnosis and management of transfusion reactions. In Clinical Practice of Transfusion Medicine, 3rd edition. Petz LD, Swisher SN, Kleinman S, Spence RK and Strauss RG eds., Churchill Livingstone, Chapter 41, 905-930, 1996

Circular of information for the use of human blood and blood components. American Association of Blood Banks, the American Red Cross, and the Council of Community Blood Centers, 1995

Brecher ME, Greenberger PA, Stack G, Judge JV, Snyder EL, Roberts GT, and Sacher RA. Tranfusion reactions. In Principles of Tranfusion Medicine, 2nd ed. Rossi EC, Simon TL, Moss GS, and Gould SA eds. Williams and Wilkins, Section XIV: Chapters 72-75, pp 747-802 1996

8g: Management of Emergent Transfusion Reactions

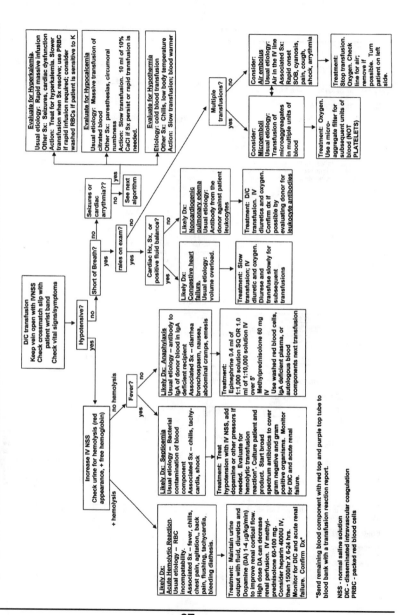

D/C transfusion
Keep vein open with IVNSS
Check crossmatch slip with patient wrist band
Check patient vital signs/symptoms

Hypotensive? yes / no

Increase IV NSS
Check urine for hemolysis (red appearance, + hemoglobin)

+ hemolysis / no hemolysis

Fever? yes / no

Short of Breath? no / yes

rales on exam? yes / no

Cardiac Hx, Sx, or positive fluid balance? yes / no

Seizures or cardiac arrythmia?? no / yes → See next algorithm

Multiple transfusions? yes / no

Likely Dx: Acute Hemolytic Reaction.
Usual etiology – RBC incompatability.
Associated Sx – fever, chills, chest pain, agitation, back pain, flushing, tachycardia, bleeding diathesis.
Treatment: Maintain urine output with fluid, diuretics and Dopamine (DA) 1-4 µg/Kg/min) to improve renal cortical flow. High dose DA can decrease renal perfusion. IV methylprednisolone 60-100 mg. Consider heparin 4000U IV, then 1500/hr X 6-24 hrs. Monitor for DIC and acute renal failure. Confirm Dx*.

Likely Dx: Septicemia
Usual etiology – Bacterial contamination of blood component
Associated Sx – chills, tachycardia, shock
Treatment: Treat hypotension with IV NSS, add dopamine or other pressors if needed. Evaluate for hemolytic transfusion reaction*. Culture patient and product. Start broad spectrum antibiotics to cover gram negative and gram positive organisms. Monitor for DIC and acute renal failure.

Likely Dx: Anaphylaxis
Usual etiology – antibody to IgA of donor blood in IgA deficient recipient
Associated Sx – diarrhea bronchospasm, nausea, abdominal cramps, emesis
Treatment:
Epinephrine 0.4 ml of 1:1,000 solution SQ OR 1.0 ml of 1:10,000 solution IV over 5'
Methylprednisolone 60 mg IV
Use washed red blood cells, IgA deficient plasma, or autologous blood components next transfusion

Likely Dx: Congestive heart failure.
Usual etiology: volume overload.
Treatment: Slow transfusion; IV diuretic and oxygen. Diurese and transfuse slowly for subsequent transfusions

Likely Dx: Noncardiogenic pulmonary edema
Usual etiology: Antibody from the donor against patient leukocytes
Treatment: D/C transfusion. IV diuretics and oxygen. Confirm dx if possible by evaluating donor for leukocyte antibodies

Evaluate for Hyperkalemia.
Usual etiology: Rapid massive infusion
Other Sx: Seizures, cardiac dysfunction
Action: Treat for hyperkalemia. Slower transfusion when Sx resolve; use PRBC if rapid infusion required; consider washed RBCs if patient is sensitive to K

Evaluate for Hypocalcemia
Usual etiology: Massive transfusion of citrated blood
Other Sx: paresthesias, circumoral numbness
Action: Slow transfusion. 10 ml of 10% CaCl if Sx persist or rapid transfusion is needed.

Evaluate for Hypothermia
Etiology: cold blood transfusion
Other Sx: Chills, low body temperature
Action: Slow transfusion; blood warmer

Consider:
Air embolism:
Usual etiology: Air in the IV line
Associated Sx: SOB, cyanosis, pain, cough, shock, arrythmia
Treatment: Stop transfusion. Oxygen. Check line for air; remove if possible. Turn patient on left side.

Consider:
Microemboli:
Usual etiology: Transfusion of microaggregates in multiple units of blood
Treatment: Oxygen. Use a micro-aggregate filter for subsequent units of blood (NOT PLATELETS)

*Send remaining blood component with red top and purple top tube to blood bank with a transfusion reaction report.

NSS - normal saline solution
DIC - disseminated intravascular coagulation
PRBC - packed red blood cells

87

9a: Nutrition equations

Ideal body weight:

Females: 100 lb (45 kg) for first 5 ft (152 cm) plus 5 lb (2.3 kg) for each additional inch (2.54 cm)
Males: 106 lbs (48 kg) for first 5 ft (152 cm) plus 6 lbs (2.7 kg) for each additional inch

Caloric requirements:

Harris - Benedict equations:

Males: $REE = 66.47 + 13.75(IBW) + 5.0H - 6.76A$
Females: $REE = 655.1 + 9.5(IBW) + 9.56H - 4.68A$

Ireton-Jones equation for obese patients: $EE = 606S + 9W - 12A + 400V + 1,444$
Ireton Jones equation for ventilator patients: $EE = 1925 - 10A + 5W + 281 S + 292T + 851B$

REE -- resting energy expenditure in kcal/day; needs to be corrected for stress. EE -- energy expenditure in kcal/day (no stress correction required). IBW -- ideal body weight (kg); H -- height in cm, A -- age in years, S -- sex (1=male, 0=female), T -- trauma (0=absent, 1 = present), B -- burn (0 = absent, 1 = present)

Weight based calculations:

Disease state	Estimate of caloric requirements
Usual maintenance diet	20-25 kcal/kg/day
Obesity (weight loss desired)	15-20 kcal/kg/day
Mild to moderate illness	25-35 kcal/kg/day
Renal disease	maintenance: 35 kcal/kg/day weight gain: 40-50 kcal/kg/day weight loss: 25-30 kcal/kg/day
Sepsis, multiorgan system failure, trauma	30-35 kcal/kg/day
Chylothorax, head trauma	35-45 kcal/kg/day
Pancreatitis, inflammatory bowel disease	45-50 kcal/kg/day

Methods of indirect calorimetry:

Weir equation for indirect calorimetry	$MEE = 1.44 (3.9 \, VO_2 + 1.1 \, VCO_2)$
Sherman equation using mixed expired CO2	$MEE = 9.27 (PECO2)(VE)$
Ligget - St. John - LeFrak equation using thermodilution cardiac output	$MEE = 95.18 (CO) (Hb) (SaO_2 - SvO_2)$

MEE = measured energy expenditure in kcal/day. VO_2 oxygen consumption in ml/min, VCO_2 -- carbon dioxide production in ml/min. $PECO_2$ -- partial pressure of expired carbon dioxide (collect several liters in nonpermeable bag, mix, withdraw 10 cc and analyze with blood gas machine); VE -- minute ventilation in liters/min. CO -- cardiac output (l/m), Hb -- hemoglobin, SaO_2 and SvO_2 are arterial and mixed venous saturations respectively.

Estimated Protein Requirements:

Minimal intake	0.54 g/day	Cancer	1.5 g/kg/day
Recommended (RDA) intake	0.80 g/day	COPD with malnutrition	1.5 - 2.0 g/kg/day
Catabolic States	1.2 - 1.6 g/kg/day	HIV infection	1 - 1.2 g/kg/day
Multiorgan system failure	1.2 - 1.5 g/kg/day (stable) 2.0 g/kg/day (stressed)	Renal disease	0.6 g/kg/day (no dialysis); increase to 1.2 (HD); 1.2-1.5 (PD); 1.5-1.8 (CAVHD)
Trauma	1.5 - 2.0 g/kg/day	Chylothorax	1.5 - 2.0 g/kg/day
Hepatic cirrhosis	1.5 g/kg/day dry weight 0.5 - 0.7 if encephalopathic	Pancreatitis/inflammatory bowel disease	1.3 - 2.0 g/kg/day

Adjust above to aim for Nitrogen Balance of +2-4 g/day: Nitrogen balance = 0.16 (g protein intake/day) - (UUN + 4)
UUN -- 24 hour urine urea nitrogen.

Fluid Requirements:

1. 35 ml/kg body weight OR
2. 1500 ml/m^2 body surface area
3. Add 150 ml/day for every degree over 37°C

Aspen Board of Directors. Guideline for the use of parenteral nutrition in adult and pediatric patients. JPEN 17(4S):7-26SA, 1993
Gottschilich MM, Matarese LE, Shronts EP. Nutrition Support Core Curriculum, Aspen Publications, 1993
Schlitig et al., Nutritional Support of the critically ill. Yearbook Medical Publishers, Chicago, 1988

9b: Nutritional Assessment and Selection of Nutritional Support Therapy

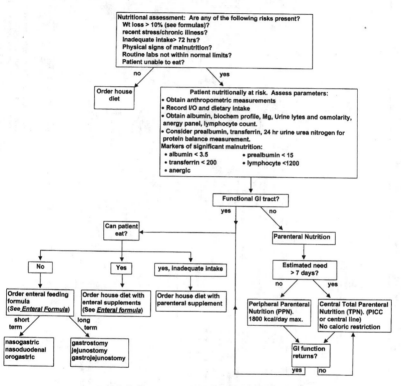

Nutritional assessment: Are any of the following risks present?
Wt loss > 10% (see formulas)?
recent stress/chronic illness?
Inadequate intake> 72 hrs?
Physical signs of malnutrition?
Routine labs not within normal limits?
Patient unable to eat?

no → Order house diet

yes → Patient nutritionally at risk. Assess parameters:
- Obtain anthropometric measurements
- Record I/O and dietary intake
- Obtain albumin, biochem profile, Mg, Urine lytes and osmolarity, anergy panel, lymphocyte count.
- Consider prealbumin, transferrin, 24 hr urine urea nitrogen for protein balance measurement.

Markers of significant malnutrition:
- albumin < 3.5
- prealbumin < 15
- transferrin < 200
- lymphocyte <1200
- anergic

Functional GI tract?

yes → Can patient eat?

no → Parenteral Nutrition → Estimated need > 7 days?

Can patient eat?
- No → Order enteral feeding formula (See *Enteral Formula*)
  - short term → nasogastric / nasoduodenal / orogastric
  - long term → gastrostomy / jejunostomy / gastrojejunostomy
- Yes → Order house diet with enteral supplements (See *Enteral formula*)
- yes, inadequate intake → Order house diet with parenteral supplement

Estimated need > 7 days?
- no → Peripheral Parenteral Nutrition (PPN). 1800 kcal/day max.
- yes → Central Total Parenteral Nutrition (TPN). (PICC or central line) No caloric restriction

GI function returns?
- yes
- no

Indications and Contraindications for Parenteral Nutrition

Indications	Contraindications
Bowel obstruction	Functioning GI tract
Ileus	Hemodynamically unstable
Hematemesis	No safe venous access
Chronic/intractable vomiting/diarrhea	Aggressive nutritional support not
Bowel rest (severe pancreatitis, chylous fistula)	warranted by prognosis
High output or Enterocutaneous fistulas	Patient does not want aggressive
Severe malabsorbtion	nutritional support
Significant catabolism and prolonged npo or clear fluid status (>5-7 days)	Treatment with TPN not anticipated for > 5 days in patients without malnutrition
Exacerbation of inflammatory bowel disease (short term)	
Short Bowel Syndrome (initially)	
Acute radiation, chemotherapy, or graft vs. host enteritis	

9c: Selecting an Enteral Formula

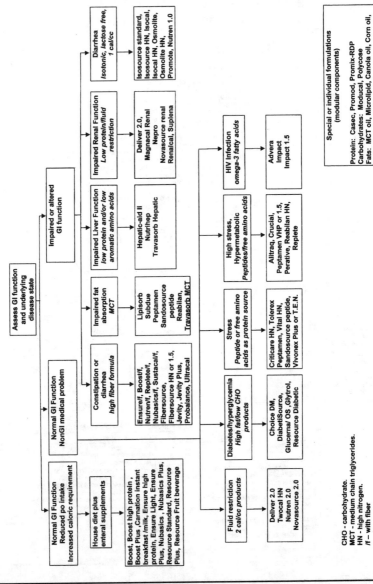

Assess GI function and underlying disease state

Normal GI Function
Reduced po intake
Increased caloric requirement

House diet plus enteral supplements

Boost, Boost high protein, Boost Plus, Carnation instant breakfast /milk, Ensure high protein, Ensure Light, Ensure Plus, Nubasics, Nubasics Plus, Resource Standard, Resource Plus, Resource Fruit beverage

Fluid restriction
2 cal/cc products

Deliver 2.0
Twocal HN
Nutren 2.0
Novasource 2.0

Normal GI Function
NonGI medical problem

Diabetes/hyperglycemia
High Fat/low CHO products

Choice DM, DiabetiSource, Glucerna/ OS, Glytrol, Resource Diabetic

Impaired or altered GI function

Constipation or diarrhea
high fiber formula

Ensure/f, Boost/f, Nutren/f, Replete/f, Nubasics/f, Sustacal/f, Fibersource, Fibersource HN or 1.5, Jevity, Jevity Plus, Probalance, Ultracal

Impaired fat absorption
MCT

Lipisorb
Subdue
Peptamen
Sandosource peptide
Reabilan, Travasorb MCT

Stress
Peptide or free amino source

Criticare HN, Tolerex, Peptamen, Vital HN, Sandosource peptide, Vivonex Plus or T.E.N.

Impaired Liver Function
low protein and/or low aromatic amino acids

Hepatic-aid II
Nutrihep
Travasorb Hepatic

Stress
Peptide or free amino acids as protein source

Alltraq, Crucial, Peptamen VHP or 1.5, Perative, Reabilan HN, Replete

Impaired Renal Function
Low protein/fluid restriction

Deliver 2.0, Magnacal Renal Nepro Novasource renal Renalcal, Suplena

High stress, Hypermetabolic
Peptides/free amino acids

Alltraq, Crucial, Peptamen VHP or 1.5, Perative, Reabilan HN, Replete

Diarrhea
Isotonic, lactose free, 1 cal/cc

Isosource standard, Isosource HN, Isocal, Isocal HN, Osmolite, Osmolite HN, Promote, Nutren 1.0

HIV Infection
omega-3 fatty acids

Advera
Impact
Impact 1.5

Special or individual formulations (modular components)

Protein: Casec, Promod, Promix-RDP
Carbohydrates: Moducal, Polycose
Fats: MCT oil, Microlipid, Canola oil, Corn oil, Safflower oil, Sunflower oil

CHO - carbohydrate.
MCT - medium chain triglycerides.
HN - high nitrogen.
/f – with fiber.

90

9d: Suggested TPN Orders

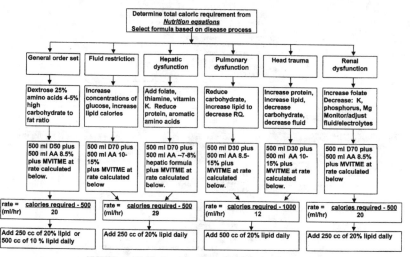

Determine total caloric requirement from
Nutrition equations
Select formula based on disease process

General order set	Fluid restriction	Hepatic dysfunction	Pulmonary dysfunction	Head trauma	Renal dysfunction
Dextrose 25% amino acids 4-5% high carbohydrate to fat ratio	Increase concentrations of glucose, increase lipid calories	Add folate, thiamine, vitamin K. Reduce protein, aromatic amino acids	Reduce carbohydrate, increase lipid to decrease RQ.	Increase protein, increase lipid, decrease carbohydrate, decrease fluid	Increase folate Decrease: K, phosphorus, Mg Monitor/adjust fluid/electrolytes
500 ml D50 plus 500 ml AA 8.5% plus MVITME at rate calculated below.	500 ml D70 plus 500 ml AA 10-15% plus MVITME at rate calculated below	500 ml D70 plus 500 ml AA ~7-8% hepatic formula plus MVITME at rate calculated below.	500 ml D30 plus 500 ml AA 8.5-15% plus MVITME at rate calculated below.	500 ml D30 plus 500 ml AA 10-15% plus MVITME at rate calculated below.	500 ml D70 plus 500 ml AA 8.5% plus MVITME at rate calculated below
rate = $\frac{calories\ required - 500}{20}$ (ml/hr)	rate = $\frac{calories\ required - 500}{29}$ (ml/hr)		rate = $\frac{calories\ required - 1000}{12}$ (ml/hr)		rate = $\frac{calories\ required - 500}{20}$ (ml/hr)
Add 250 cc of 20% lipid or 500 cc of 10 % lipid daily	Add 250 cc of 20% lipid daily		Add 500 cc of 20% lipid daily		Add 250 cc of 20% lipid daily

MVITME -- multivitamins, trace elements, minerals, electrolytes

Vitamin	IV Dose/day	Additive	IV dose	Trace elements	IV dose/day
Vit A	3300 IU	Cobalamin (B12)	5.0 µg/day	Chromium	10-15 mcg
Vit C	200 IU	Ascorbic acid (C)	100 mg/day	Copper	0.05-1.5 mg
Vit E	10 IU	Vit K*	2.5 mg/day	Iodine	1-2 mcg/kg
Thiamine (B1)	3.0 mg	Potassium[1]	60-100 mEq/l	Manganese	0.15-0.8 mg
Riboflavin (B2)	3.6 mg	Sodium[1]	60-130 mEq/l	Selenium	30-200 mcg
Niacin (B3)	15.0 mg	Acetate[2]	0--130 mEq/l	Zinc[3]	2.5-4.0 mg
Pantothenic acid (B5)	40.0 mg	Calcium[1]	5-15 mEq/l	Iron	1-2.5 mg
Pyridoxine (B6)	4.0 mg	Phosphorus[1]	15-45 mEq/l	Molybdenum	20 mcg
Biotin (B7)	60.0 mg	Magnesium[1]	10-30 mEq/l		
Floacin (B9)	400.0 µg	Chloride[1]	60-130 mEq/l		

*Vitamin K can be given as 10 mg weekly; do not give to patients on coumadin

1. check serum levels and adjust. Sodium is usually given as NaCl. Add (or replace NaCl with) Na acetate starting at 40 mEq/liter if serum CO2 < 25 meq/liter and adjust based on serum CO2 response. Do not exceed 150 mEq Na/l
 • Add K as KCl if serum CO2>25mEq/l; add K as K acetate if serum CO2 < 25 mEq/l.
 • Calcium is usually given as Ca gluconate. Add 9 mEq/l if serum Ca < 8.5 meq/l; add 4.5 mEq/l if serum Ca > 8.5 meq/l.; do not exceed 27 mEq/day.
2. Use for correction of acidosis in patients without hepatic dysfunction. May give as Na acetate or K acetate. K acetate should not exceed 40 meq/l.
3. Additional zinc may be required in acute catabolism (2mg/day), small bowel fluid losses (12.2 mg/liter fluid loss), and diarrhea/ileostomy output (17.1 mg/kg of output)

Nutritional values of intravenous sources

Solution	Kcal/Liter	Solution	kcal/cc	kcal/250 ml	crystalline amino acids	grams/liter
5% dextrose	170	10 % lipid	1.1	275	5.5%	55
10% dextrose	340	20% lipid	2.0	500	8.5%	85
30% dextrose	1020	30% lipid	3.0	750	10%	100
50% dextrose	1700				15%	150
70% dextrose	2380				8.0% hepatic	80

Grant J. Handbook of Total Parenteral Nutrition, 2nd ed. WB Saunders, Phila, PA, 1992.
Sheldon et. al., Electrolyte requirements in total parenteral nutrition. in Nutrition in Clinical Surgery, Dietel M (ed), 1985
Schlitig et al. Nutritional Support of the Critically Ill. Yearbook Medical Publishers, Chicago 1988

10a: Hyponatremia

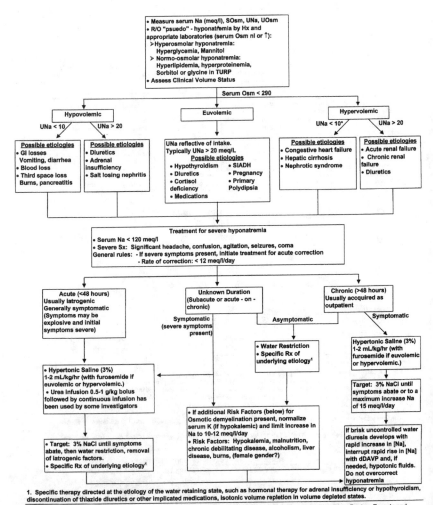

- Measure serum Na (meq/l), SOsm, UNa, UOsm
- R/O "psuedo" - hyponatremia by Hx and appropriate laboratories (serum Osm nl or ↑):
  - ➤ Hyperosmolar hyponatremia: Hyperglycemia, Mannitol
  - ➤ Normo-osmolar hyponatremia: Hyperlipidemia, hyperproteinemia, Sorbitol or glycine in TURP
- Assess Clinical Volume Status

Serum Osm < 290

Hypovolemic — UNa < 10 / UNa > 20

Euvolemic

Hypervolemic — UNa < 10* / UNa > 20

Possible etiologies
- GI losses Vomiting, diarrhea
- Blood loss
- Third space loss Burns, pancreatitis

Possible etiologies
- Diuretics
- Adrenal insufficiency
- Salt losing nephritis

UNa reflective of intake. Typically UNa > 20 meq/L.
Possible etiologies
- Hypothyroidism
- Diuretics
- Cortisol deficiency
- Medications
- SIADH
- Pregnancy
- Primary Polydipsia

Possible etiologies
- Congestive heart failure
- Hepatic cirrhosis
- Nephrotic syndrome

Possible etiologies
- Acute renal failure
- Chronic renal failure
- Diuretics

Treatment for severe hyponatremia
- Serum Na < 120 meq/l
- Severe Sx: Significant headache, confusion, agitation, seizures, coma
- General rules: - If severe symptoms present, initiate treatment for acute correction
  - Rate of correction: < 12 meq/l/day

Acute (<48 hours)
Usually iatrogenic
Generally symptomatic
(Symptoms may be explosive and initial symptoms severe)

Unknown Duration
(Subacute or acute - on - chronic)
Symptomatic (severe symptoms present) / Asymptomatic

Chronic (>48 hours)
Usually acquired as outpatient
Symptomatic

- Hypertonic Saline (3%) 1-2 mL/kg/hr (with furosemide if euvolemic or hypervolemic.)
- Urea infusion 0.5-1 g/kg bolus followed by continuous infusion has been used by some investigators

- Water Restriction
- Specific Rx of underlying etiology[1]

Hypertonic Saline (3%) 1-2 mL/kg/hr (with furosemide if euvolemic or hypervolemic.)

- Target: 3% NaCl until symptoms abate, then water restriction, removal of iatrogenic factors.
- Specific Rx of underlying etiology[1]

- If additional Risk Factors (below) for Osmotic demyelination present, normalize serum K (if hypokalemic) and limit increase in Na to 10-12 meq/l/day
- Risk Factors: Hypokalemia, malnutrition, chronic debilitating disease, alcoholism, liver disease, burns, (female gender?)

Target: 3% NaCl until symptoms abate or to a maximum increase Na of 15 meq/l/day

If brisk uncontrolled water diuresis develops with rapid increase in [Na], interrupt rapid rise in [Na] with dDAVP and, if needed, hypotonic fluids. Do not overcorrect hyponatremia

1. Specific therapy directed at the etiology of the water retaining state, such as hormonal therapy for adrenal insufficiency or hypothyroidism, discontinuation of thiazide diuretics or other implicated medications, isotonic volume repletion in volume depleted states.

Beri T, Schreier RW. Disorders of water metabolism. In Schrier editor: Renal and Electrolyte Disorders 4th edition, Boston, Toronto and London, Little Brown and Company 1992
Soupart A, Decaux G. Therapeutic recommendations for management of severe hyponatremia. Clinical Nephrology 46: 149-169, 1996

10b: Hypernatremia

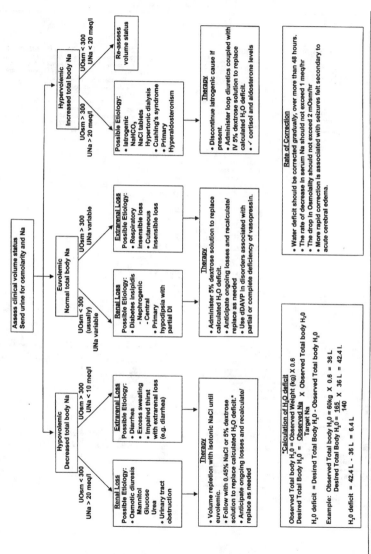

Assess clinical volume status
Send urine for osmolarity and Na

Hypovolemic
Decreased total body Na

Renal Loss
UOsm < 300
UNa > 20 meq/l
Possible Etiology:
- Osmotic diuresis
  Mannitol
  Glucose
  Urea
- Urinary tract obstruction

Extrarenal Loss
UOsm > 300
UNa < 10 meq/l
Possible Etiology:
- Diarrhea
- Excess sweating
- Impaired thirst with extrarenal loss (e.g. diarrhea)

Therapy
- Volume repletion with isotonic NaCl until euvolemic.
- Follow with 0.45% NaCl or 5% dextrose solution to replace calculated H₂O deficit.*
- Anticipate ongoing losses and recalculate/replace as needed

Euvolemic
Normal total body Na

Renal Loss
UOsm < 300 (usually)
UNa variable
Possible Etiology:
- Diabetes insipidis
  - Nephrogenic
  - Central
- Primary hypodipsia with partial DI

Extrarenal Loss
UOsm > 300
UNa variable
Possible Etiology:
- Respiratory insensible loss
- Cutaneous insensible loss

Therapy
- Administer 5% dextrose solution to replace calculated H₂O deficit.
- Anticipate ongoing losses and recalculate/replace as needed
- Use dDAVP in disorders associated with partial or complete deficiency of vasopressin.

Hypervolemic
Increased total body Na

UOsm > 300
UNa > 20 meq/l
Possible Etiology:
- Iatrogenic
  NaHCO₃
  NaCl tablets
  Hypertonic dialysis
- Cushing's syndrome
- Primary Hyperaldosteronism

UOsm < 300
UNa < 20 meq/l
Re-assess volume status

Therapy
- Discontinue iatrogenic cause if present.
- Administer loop diuretics coupled with IV 5% dextrose solution to replace calculated H₂O deficit.
- ✓ cortisol and aldosterone levels

Rate of Correction
- Water deficit should be corrected *gradually*, over more than 48 hours.
- The rate of decrease in serum Na should not exceed 1 meq/hr
- The drop in Osmolality should not exceed 2 mOsm/hr
- More rapid correction is associated with seizures felt secondary to acute cerebral edema.

*Calculation of H₂O deficit

Observed Total body H_2O = Observed Weight (kg) X 0.6

Desired Total Body H_2O = $\dfrac{\text{Observed Total Body } H_2O \text{ X Observed Total body } H_2O}{\text{Target Na}}$

H_2O deficit = Desired Total Body H_2O - Observed Total body H_2O

Example: Observed Total body H_2O = 60kg X 0.6 = 36 L

Desired Total Body H_2O = $\dfrac{165}{140}$ X 36 L = 42.4 L.

H_2O deficit = 42.4 L - 36 L = 6.4 L

Beri T, Schreier RW. Disorders of water metabolism. In Schrier editor: Renal and Electrolyte Disorders 4th edition, Boston, Toronto and London,k Little Brown and Company 1992
Sterns RH, Spital A. Disorders of water balance. In Kokko, Tannen editors: Fluid and Electrolytes, Philadelphia, WB Saunders, 1990.

10c: Hyperkalemia

(Serum $K^+ > 5.5$ mEq/L)

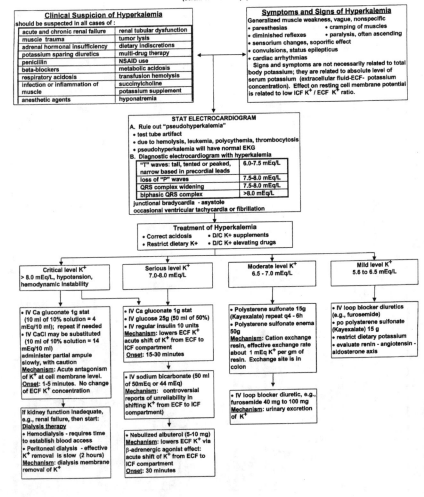

Clinical Suspicion of Hyperkalemia

should be suspected in all cases of :

acute and chronic renal failure	renal tubular dysfunction
muscle trauma	tumor lysis
adrenal hormonal insufficiency	dietary indiscretions
potassium sparing diuretics	multi-drug therapy
penicillin	NSAID use
beta-blockers	metabolic acidosis
respiratory acidosis	transfusion hemolysis
infection or inflammation of muscle	succinylcholine
	potassium supplement
anesthetic agents	hyponatremia

Symptoms and Signs of Hyperkalemia

Generalized muscle weakness, vague, nonspecific
- paresthesias
- cramping of muscles
- diminished reflexes
- paralysis, often ascending
- sensorium changes, soporific effect
- convulsions, status epilepticus
- cardiac arrhythmias

Signs and symptoms are not necessarily related to total body potassium; they are related to absolute level of serum potassium (extracellular fluid-ECF- potassium concentration). Effect on resting cell membrane potential is related to low ICF K^+ / ECF K^+ ratio.

STAT ELECTROCARDIOGRAM

A. Rule out "pseudohyperkalemia"
- test tube artifact
- due to hemolysis, leukemia, polycythemia, thrombocytosis
- pseudohyperkalemia will have normal EKG

B. Diagnostic electrocardiogram with hyperkalemia

"T" waves: tall, tented or peaked, narrow based in precordial leads	6.0-7.5 mEq/L
loss of "P" waves	7.5-8.0 mEq/L
QRS complex widening	7.5-8.0 mEq/L
biphasic QRS complex	>8.0 mEq/L

junctional bradycardia - asystole
occasional ventricular tachycardia or fibrillation

Treatment of Hyperkalemia

- Correct acidosis
- D/C K+ supplements
- Restrict dietary K+
- D/C K+ elevating drugs

Critical level K^+
> 8.0 mEq/L, hypotension, hemodynamic instability

- IV Ca gluconate 1g stat (10 ml of 10% solution = 4 mEq/10 ml); repeat if needed
- IV CaCl may be substituted (10 ml of 10% solution = 14 mEq/10 ml)
administer partial ampule slowly, with caution
Mechanism: Acute antagonism of K^+ at cell membrane level.
Onset: 1-5 minutes. No change of ECF K^+ concentration

If kidney function inadequate, e.g., renal failure, then start:
Dialysis therapy
- Hemodialysis - requires time to establish blood access
- Peritoneal dialysis - effective K^+ removal is slow (2 hours)
Mechanism: dialysis membrane removal of K^+

Serious level K^+
7.0-8.0 mEq/L

- IV Ca gluconate 1g stat
- IV glucose 25g (50 ml of 50%)
- IV regular insulin 10 units
Mechanism: lowers ECF K^+ acute shift of K^+ from ECF to ICF compartment
Onset: 15-30 minutes

- IV sodium bicarbonate (50 ml of 50mEq or 44 mEq)
Mechanism: controversial reports of unreliability in shifting K^+ from ECF to ICF compartment)

- Nebulized albuterol (5-10 mg)
Mechanism: lowers ECF K^+ via β-adrenergic agonist effect: acute shift of K^+ from ECF to ICF compartment
Onset: 30 minutes

Moderate level K^+
6.5 - 7.0 mEq/L

- Polysterene sulfonate 15g (Kayexalate) repeat q4 - 6h
- Polysterene sulfonate enema 50g
Mechanism: Cation exchange resin, effective exchange rate about 1 mEq K^+ per gm of resin. Exchange site is in colon

- IV loop blocker diuretic, e.g., furosemide 40 mg to 100 mg
Mechanism: urinary excretion of K^+

Mild level K^+
5.6 to 6.5 mEq/L

- IV loop blocker diuretics (e.g., furosemide)
- po polysterene sulfonate (Kayexalate) 15 g
- restrict dietary potassium
- evaluate renin - angiotensin - aldosterone axis

10d: Hypokalemia

(serum K^+ < 3.5 mEq/L)

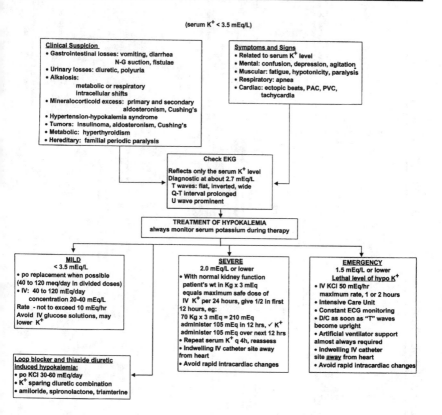

Clinical Suspicion
- Gastrointestinal losses: vomiting, diarrhea
  - N-G suction, fistulae
- Urinary losses: diuretic, polyuria
- Alkalosis:
  - metabolic or respiratory
  - intracellular shifts
- Mineralocorticoid excess: primary and secondary
  - aldosteronism, Cushing's
- Hypertension-hypokalemia syndrome
- Tumors: insulinoma, aldosteronism, Cushing's
- Metabolic: hyperthyroidism
- Hereditary: familial periodic paralysis

Symptoms and Signs
- Related to serum K^+ level
- Mental: confusion, depression, agitation
- Muscular: fatigue, hypotonicity, paralysis
- Respiratory: apnea
- Cardiac: ectopic beats, PAC, PVC,
  - tachycardia

Check EKG

Reflects only the serum K^+ level
Diagnostic at about 2.7 mEq/L
T waves: flat, inverted, wide
Q-T interval prolonged
U wave prominent

TREATMENT OF HYPOKALEMIA
always monitor serum potassium during therapy

MILD
< 3.5 mEq/L
- po replacement when possible
  (40 to 120 meq/day in divided doses)
- IV: 40 to 120 mEq/day
  concentration 20-40 mEq/L
  Rate - not to exceed 10 mEq/hr
  Avoid IV glucose solutions, may
  lower K^+

SEVERE
2.0 mEq/L or lower
- With normal kidney function
  patient's wt in Kg x 3 mEq
  equals maximum safe dose of
  IV K^+ per 24 hours, give 1/2 in first
  12 hours, eg:
  70 Kg x 3 mEq = 210 mEq
  administer 105 mEq in 12 hrs, ✓ K^+
  administer 105 mEq over next 12 hrs
- Repeat serum K^+ q 4h, reassess
- Indwelling IV catheter site away
  from heart
- Avoid rapid intracardiac changes

EMERGENCY
1.5 mEq/L or lower
Lethal level of hypo K^+
- IV KCl 50 mEq/hr
  maximum rate, 1 or 2 hours
- Intensive Care Unit
- Constant ECG monitoring
- D/C as soon as "T" waves
  become upright
- Artificial ventilator support
  almost always required
- Indwelling IV catheter
  site away from heart
- Avoid rapid intracardiac changes

Loop blocker and thiazide diuretic
induced hypokalemia:
- po KCl 30-60 mEq/day
- K^+ sparing diuretic combination
- amiloride, spironolactone, triamterine

Most cases require potassium replacement as KCl especially if alkalosis co-exists
In cases of metabolic acidosis, consider using K acetate, gluconate, or citrate (bicarbonate precursors)

10e: Evaluation and Management of Hypocalcemia

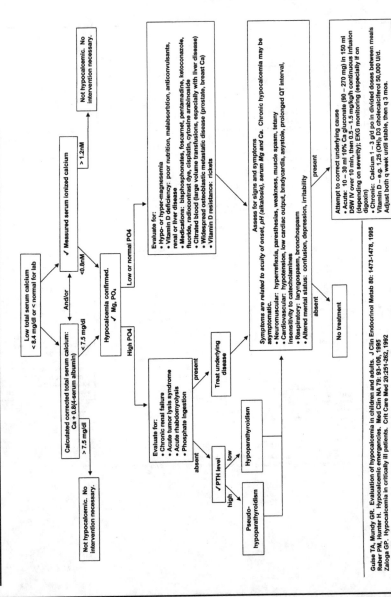

Guise TA, Mundy GR. Evaluation of hypocalcemia in children and adults. J Clin Endocrinol Metab 80: 1473-1478, 1995
Reber PM, Hunter H. Hypocalcemic emergencies. Med Clin NA 79: 93-106, 1995
Zaloga GP. Hypocalcemia in critically ill patients. Crit Care Med 20:251-262, 1992

10f: Evaluation and Management of Hypercalcemia

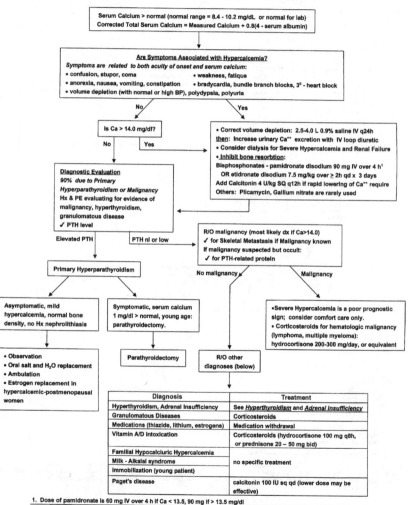

Serum Calcium > normal (normal range = 8.4 - 10.2 mg/dL or normal for lab)
Corrected Total Serum Calcium = Measured Calcium + 0.8(4 - serum albumin)

Are Symptoms Associated with Hypercalcemia?
Symptoms are related to both acuity of onset and serum calcium:
- confusion, stupor, coma
- anorexia, nausea, vomiting, constipation
- volume depletion (with normal or high BP), polydypsia, polyuria
- weakness, fatigue
- bradycardia, bundle branch blocks, 3° - heart block

No → Is Ca > 14.0 mg/dl?

Yes →
- Correct volume depletion: 2.5-4.0 L 0.9% saline IV q24h
  <u>then</u>: Increase urinary Ca^{++} excretion with IV loop diuretic
- Consider dialysis for Severe Hypercalcemia and Renal Failure
- <u>Inhibit bone resorption:</u>
  Bisphosphonates - pamidronate disodium 90 mg IV over 4 h[1]
  OR etidronate disodium 7.5 mg/kg over ≥ 2h qd x 3 days
  Add Calcitonin 4 U/kg SQ q12h if rapid lowering of Ca^{++} require
  Others: Plicamycin, Gallium nitrate are rarely used

Diagnostic Evaluation
90% due to Primary Hyperparathyroidism or Malignancy
Hx & PE evaluating for evidence of malignancy, hyperthyroidism, granulomatous disease
✓ PTH level

Elevated PTH → **Primary Hyperparathyroidism**

PTH nl or low →

R/O malignancy (most likely dx if Ca>14.0)
✓ for Skeletal Metastasis if Malignancy known
If malignancy suspected but occult:
✓ for PTH-related protein

No malignancy / Malignancy

Asymptomatic, mild hypercalcemia, normal bone density, no Hx nephrolithiasis
- Observation
- Oral salt and H$_2$O replacement
- Ambulation
- Estrogen replacement in hypercalcemic-postmenopausal women

Symptomatic, serum calcium 1 mg/dl > normal, young age: parathyroidectomy.
→ Parathyroidectomy

R/O other diagnoses (below)

- Severe Hypercalcemia is a poor prognostic sign; consider comfort care only.
- Corticosteroids for hematologic malignancy (lymphoma, multiple myeloma): hydrocortisone 200-300 mg/day, or equivalent

Diagnosis	Treatment
Hyperthyroidism, Adrenal Insufficiency	See *Hyperthyroidism* and *Adrenal Insufficiency*
Granulomatous Diseases	Corticosteroids
Medications (thiazide, lithium, estrogens)	Medication withdrawal
Vitamin A/D Intoxication	Corticosteroids (hydrocortisone 100 mg q8h, or prednisone 20 – 50 mg bid)
Familial Hypocalciuric Hypercalcemia	
Milk - Alkalai syndrome	no specific treatment
Immobilization (young patient)	
Paget's disease	calcitonin 100 IU sq qd (lower dose may be effective)

1. Dose of pamidronate is 60 mg IV over 4 h if Ca < 13.5, 90 mg if > 13.5 mg/dl

Bilezikian JP. Management of Hypercalcemia. J Clin Endocrinol Metab 77:1445, 1993.
Edelson GW, Kleerekoper M. Hypercalcemic Crisis Med Clin North Am 79:79, 1995.

11a: Initial Diagnostic Approach to Acute Low Back Pain

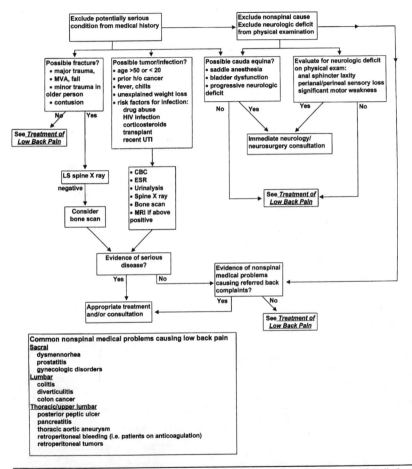

Common nonspinal medical problems causing low back pain

Sacral
- dysmennorhea
- prostatitis
- gynecologic disorders

Lumbar
- colitis
- diverticulitis
- colon cancer

Thoracic/upper lumbar
- posterior peptic ulcer
- pancreatitis
- thoracic aortic aneurysm
- retroperitoneal bleeding (i.e. patients on anticoagulation)
- retroperitoneal tumors

Bigos S, Bowyer O, Braen G, et al. Acute Low Back Problems in Adults. Clinical Practice Guideline, Quick Reference Guide Number. 14. Rockville, MD: U.S. Department of Health and Human Services, Public Health Service, Agency for Health Care Policy and Research, AHCPR Pub. No. 95-0643, December 1994.

11b: Treatment of Low Back Pain

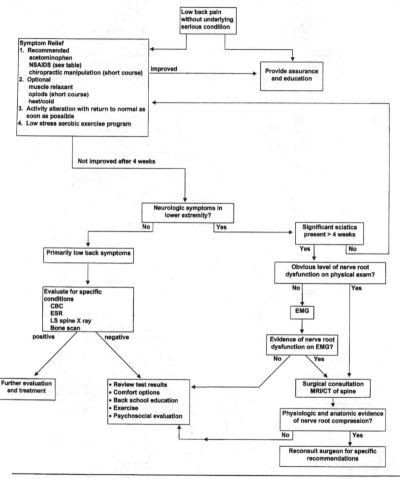

Bigos S, Bowyer O, Braen G, et al. Acute Low Back Problems in Adults. Clinical Practice Guideline, Quick Reference Guide Number. 14. Rockville, MD: U.S. Department of Health and Human Services, Public Health Service, Agency for Health Care Policy and Research, AHCPR Pub. No. 95-0643, December 1994.

11c: Differential Diagnosis and Management of Acute Monoarthritis

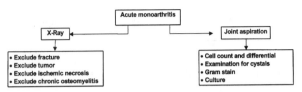

Types of Joint effusions

Criteria	Normal	Non-inflammatory	Inflammatory	Purulent	Hemorrhagic
1. volume	<3.5 ml	often >3.5 ml	often >3.5 ml	>3.5 ml	>3.5 ml
2. color	clear	xanthochromic	xanthochromic to white	depends on organism	bloody
3. clarity	transparent	transparent	translucent to opaque	opaque	bloody
4. viscosity	high	high	low	variable	like blood
5. mucin clot	firm	firm	friable	friable	
6. clot	no	occasional	often	often	
7. WBC(mm3)	<200	200-2000	2000-100,000 (20,000 average)	>50,000	blood
8. % polys	<25%	<25%	>75%	>75%	blood
9. culture	Neg	Neg	Neg	Pos or Neg	Neg

Differential Diagnosis of Joint Effusions

Non-inflammatory	Inflammatory	Purulent	Hemorrhagic
Osteoarthritis	Rheumatoid arthritis	Bacterial infection	Trauma
Trauma	Reiter's syndrome	Acute gout	Fracture
Osteochondritis	Acute crystal synovitis		Blood dyscrasia
Avascular necrosis	Psoriatic arthritis		Charcot joint
SLE	Enteropathic arthritis		Pigmented villonodular synovitis
Amyloidosis	Lyme Disease		Tumor
Chronic crystal synovitis	Viral arthritis		
	Rheumatic fever		
	Infectious arthritis		
	bacterial		
	tuberculosis		
	fungal		

Aspiration of Inflammatory or Purulent Fluid from Monoarthritis

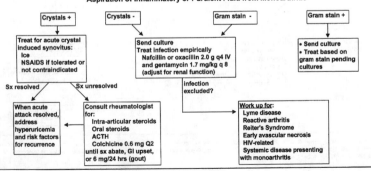

1. Baker, DG and Schumacher, HR. Acute Monoarthritis. NEJM 329:1013-1020, 1993.
2. Emmerson, BT. The Management of Gout. NEJM. 334:445-451, 1996.

11d: Medical Management of Osteoarthritis of the Hip and Knee

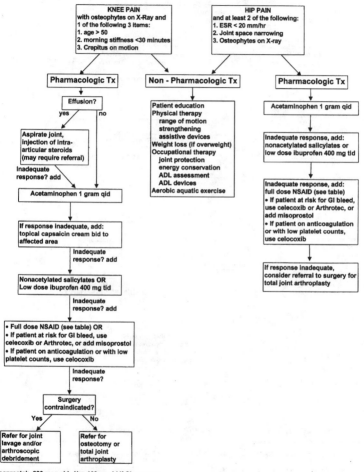

KNEE PAIN
with osteophytes on X-Ray and
1 of the following 3 items:
1. age > 50
2. morning stiffness <30 minutes
3. Crepitus on motion

HIP PAIN
and at least 2 of the following:
1. ESR < 20 mm/hr
2. Joint space narrowing
3. Osteophytes on X-ray

Pharmacologic Tx

Effusion?

yes   no

Aspirate joint,
injection of intra-
articular steroids
(may require referral)

Inadequate
response? add

Acetaminophen 1 gram qid

If response inadequate, add:
topical capsaicin cream bid to
affected area

Inadequate
response? add

Nonacetylated salicylates OR
Low dose ibuprofen 400 mg tid

Inadequate
response? add

• Full dose NSAID (see table) OR
• If patient at risk for GI bleed, use
celecoxib or Arthrotec, or add misoprostol
• If patient on anticoagulation or with low
platelet counts, use celocoxib

Inadequate
response?

Surgery
contraindicated?

Yes   No

Refer for joint
lavage and/or
arthroscopic
debridement

Refer for
osteotomy or
total joint
arthroplasty

Non - Pharmacologic Tx

Patient education
Physical therapy
    range of motion
    strengthening
    assistive devices
Weight loss (if overweight)
Occupational therapy
    joint protection
    energy conservation
    ADL assessment
    ADL devices
Aerobic aquatic exercise

Pharmacologic Tx

Acetaminophen 1 gram qid

Inadequate response, add:
nonacetylated salicylates or
low dose ibuprofen 400 mg tid

Inadequate response, add:
full dose NSAID (see table)
• If patient at risk for GI bleed,
use celecoxib or Arthrotec, or
add misoprostol
• If patient on anticoagulation
or with low platelet counts,
use celecoxib

If response inadequate,
consider referral to surgery for
total joint arthroplasty

misoprostol: 200 mcg qid. Use 100mg qid if GI sx occur.
*Risk factors for GI bleed: age >75, h/o peptic ulcer diseae, GI bleed, or heart disease.

1. Hochberg, MC. et al. Guidelines for the Medical Management of Osteoarthritis. Part I. Osteoarthritis of the Hip. Arthritis Rheum. 38:1535-1549, 1995
2. Hochberg, MC. et al. Guidelines for the Medical Management of Osteoarthritis. Part II. Osteoarthritis of the Knee. Arthritis Rheum. 38:1541-1546, 1995.

11e: Differential Diagnosis of Polyarthritis

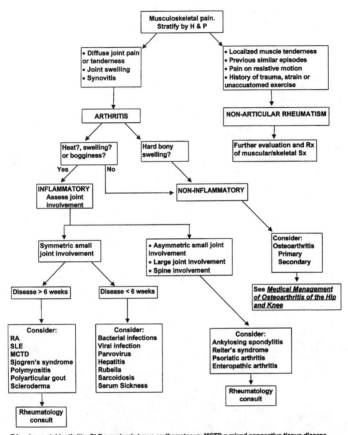

RA = rheumatoid arthritis; SLE = systemic lupus erythematosus; MCTD = mixed connective tissue disease

1. Sergent, JS. Polyarticular Arthritis. Chapter 23 in Kelley, WN. Textbook of Rheumatology. 4th Edition, W.B. Saunders Company, pp381-388, 1993.
2. Pinals, RS. Polyarthritis and Fever. NEJM. 330:769-774, 1994.
3. Rheumatologic Disorders: An Office Guide to Differential Diagnosis. Syntex Laboratories Inc. Issue 10, June 1979.

11f: Medical Management of Rheumatoid Arthritis

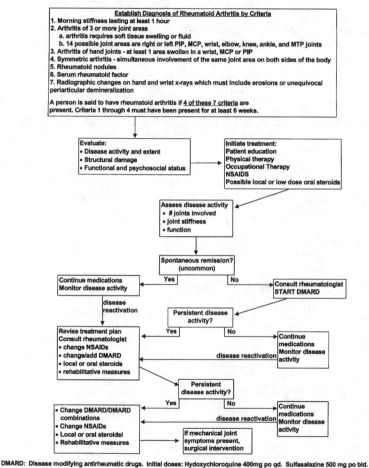

Establish Diagnosis of Rheumatoid Arthritis by Criteria
1. Morning stiffness lasting at least 1 hour
2. Arthritis of 3 or more joint areas
   a. arthritis requires soft tissue swelling or fluid
   b. 14 possible joint areas are right or left PIP, MCP, wrist, elbow, knee, ankle, and MTP joints
3. Arthritis of hand joints - at least 1 area swollen in a wrist, MCP or PIP
4. Symmetric arthritis - simultaneous involvement of the same joint area on both sides of the body
5. Rheumatoid nodules
6. Serum rheumatoid factor
7. Radiographic changes on hand and wrist x-rays which must include erosions or unequivocal periarticular demineralization

A person is said to have rheumatoid arthritis if 4 of these 7 criteria are present. Criteria 1 through 4 must have been present for at least 6 weeks.

Evaluate:
- Disease activity and extent
- Structural damage
- Functional and psychosocial status

Initiate treatment:
Patient education
Physical therapy
Occupational Therapy
NSAIDS
Possible local or low dose oral steroids

Assess disease activity
- # joints involved
- joint stiffness
- function

Spontaneous remission?
(uncommon)

Continue medications
Monitor disease activity

Yes   No   Consult rheumatologist
                 START DMARD

disease reactivation

Persistent disease activity?

Revise treatment plan
Consult rheumatologist
- change NSAIDs
- change/add DMARD
- local or oral steroids
- rehabilitative measures

Yes   No   Continue medications
                 Monitor disease activity
         disease reactivation

Persistent disease activity?

- Change DMARD/DMARD combinations
- Change NSAIDs
- Local or oral steroids!
- Rehabilitative measures

Yes   No   Continue medications
                 Monitor disease activity
         disease reactivation

If mechanical joint symptoms present, surgical intervention

DMARD: Disease modifying antirheumatic drugs. Initial doses: Hydoxychloroquine 400mg po qd. Sulfasalazine 500 mg po bid. Methotrexate 7.5 mg po or SC weekly. Leflunomide 100 mg po qd for 3 days, then 20 mg qd. Etanercept 25 mg SC twice weekly. Gold salts 10 mg test dose, then 50 mg weekly. Auranofin 3 mg po BID. Penicillamine 250 mg qd. Minocin 100 mg po bid. All DMARDs should be prescribed by physicians familiar with their use and many require specific monitoring.

1. Arnett, FC. et al. The American Rheumatism Association 1987 Revised Criteria for the Classification of Rheumatoid Arthritis. Arthritis Rheum. 31:315-324, 1988
2. American College of Rheumatology Ad Hoc Committee on Clinical Guidelines. Guidelines for the Management of Rheumatoid Arthritis. Arthritis Rheum. 39:713-722, 1996.

11g: Table of Nonsteroidal Anti-Inflammatory Drugs (NSAIDs)

Salicylates

Generic	Brand name	Dose Range (mg/day)*	Dose Interval	Comments
Acetylsalicylic acid	Aspirin	1000-6000	q.i.d.	

Nonacetylated salicylates

Generic	Brand name	Dose Range (mg/day)*	Dose Interval	Comments
Choline magnesium trisalicylate	Trilisate	1500-3000	b.i.d. to t.i.d.	Liquid available Salicylate levels available
Salicylsalicylic acid	Disalcid	1500-3000	b.i.d. to t.i.d.	Salicylate levels available
	Salflex	1500-3000	b.i.d. to t.i.d.	Salicylate levels available

Nonacetylated salicylates have decreased effects on platelets, gastric mucosa and prostaglandin mediated renal function as compared to acetylsalicylic acid. They are generally considered safe in aspirin-sensitive asthma.

Short Serum Half Life NSAIDs

Generic	Brand name	Dose Range (mg/day)*	Dose Interval	Comments
Diclofenac potassium	Cataflam	100-200	bid to tid	Monitor ALT (SGPT) within
Diclofenac sodium	Voltaran	100-200	bid to tid	4 – 8 weeks
Fenoprofen calcium	Nalfon	1200-3200	tid to qid	Acute interstitial nephritis
Flurbiprofen	Ansaid	100-300	bid to qid	
Ibuprofen	Motrin	1200-3200	tid to qid	Liquid available
Ketoprofen	Orudis	150-300	tid to qid	
	Oruvail	150-300	qd	
Meclofenamate sodium	Meclomen	200-400	tid to qid	Higher incidence of diarrhea
Tolmetin sodium	Tolectin	800-1800	tid	Pediatric approval for JRA

Long Serum Half Life NSAIDs

Generic	Brand name	Dose Range (mg/day)*	Dose Interval	Comments
Diflunisal	Dolobid	500-1500	bid	A derivative of salicylate but not metabolized to salicylate.
Indomethacin	Indocin	50-200	bid to tid	Efficacy in ankylosing spondylitis and gout
Nabumetone	Relafen	1000-2000	qd to bid	Nonacidic pro-drug undergoes hepatic transformation to active acidic metabolite. Liver function abnormalities. Use with care in liver disease
Naproxen sodium	Naprosyn	750-1500	bid	Liquid available Pediatric approval for JRA
Oxaprozin	Daypro	600-1200	qd	
Piroxicam	Feldene	20	qd	
Sulindac	Clinoril	300-400	bid	May have a lower incidence of prostaglandin-mediated renal effects.

Cox-2 specific NSAIDS

Generic	Brand name	Dose Range (mg/day)*	Dose Interval	Comments
Celecoxib	Celebrex	200-400	qd to bid	No effect on platelet function. Decreased GI side effects. Contraindicated if sulfonamide allergy

*Doses are given as mg/day and should be divided by the dose interval when prescribing

1. Borigini, MJ and Paulus, HE. Rheumatoid Arthritis. in Weisman, MH and Weinblatt, ME. Treatment of the Rheumatic Diseases, W.B. Saunders Co.,pp 31-51, 1995
2. Physician's Desk Reference. Medical Economics Data Production Company, 1999.

11h: Evaluation of Suspected Vasculitis

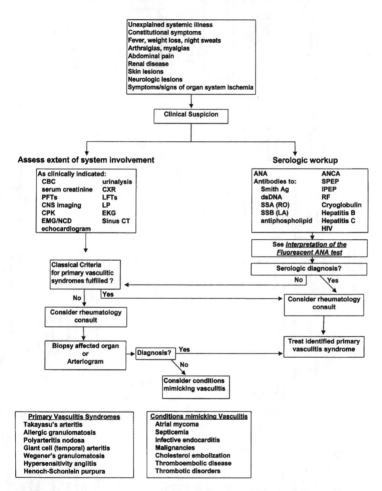

Unexplained systemic illness
Constitutional symptoms
Fever, weight loss, night sweats
Arthralgias, myalgias
Abdominal pain
Renal disease
Skin lesions
Neurologic lesions
Symptoms/signs of organ system ischemia

Clinical Suspicion

Assess extent of system involvement

As clinically indicated:
CBC	urinalysis
serum creatinine	CXR
PFTs	LFTs
CNS imaging	LP
CPK	EKG
EMG/NCD	Sinus CT
echocardiogram	

Serologic workup

ANA	ANCA
Antibodies to:	SPEP
Smith Ag	IPEP
dsDNA	RF
SSA (RO)	Cryoglobulin
SSB (LA)	Hepatitis B
antiphospholipid	Hepatitis C
	HIV

See *Interpretation of the Fluorescent ANA test*

Serologic diagnosis?   No   Yes

Classical Criteria for primary vasculitic syndromes fulfilled ?

No   Yes

Consider rheumatology consult

Consider rheumatology consult

Biopsy affected organ or Arteriogram   Diagnosis?   Yes   No

Treat identified primary vasculitis syndrome

Consider conditions mimicking vasculitis

Primary Vasculitis Syndromes	**Conditions mimicking Vasculitis**
Takayasu's arteritis	Atrial mycoma
Allergic granulomatosis	Septicemia
Polyarteritis nodosa	Infective endocarditis
Giant cell (temporal) arteritis	Malignancies
Wegener's granulomatosis	Cholesterol embolization
Hypersensitivity angiitis	Thromboembolic disease
Henoch-Schonlein purpura	Thrombotic disorders

ANA - antinuclear antibody. dsDNA - double stranded DNA. RNP - ribonuclear protein. HIV-human immune deficiency virus. SPEP-serum protein electrophoresis. IPEP - immune protein electrophoresis. RF - rheumatoid factor. NCV-nerve conduction velocities

Conn, DL et al. Vasculitis and Related Disorders. In Kelly WN ed, Textbook of Rheumatology, WB Saunders, pp. 1077-1102, 1993

11i: Interpretation of the Fluorescent Antinuclear Antibody Test

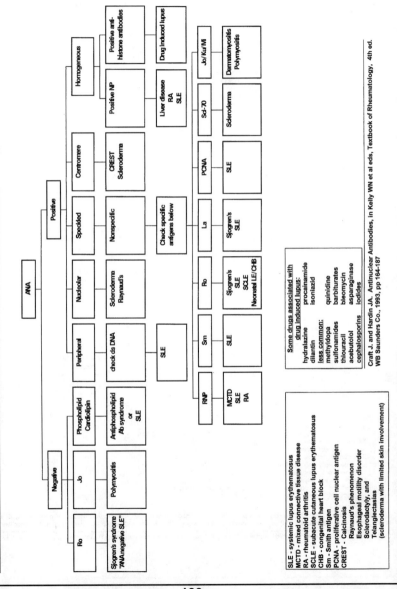

Craft J. and Hardin JA. Antinuclear Antibodies, in Kelly WN et al eds, Textbook of Rheumatology, 4th ed. WB Saunders Co., 1993, pp 164-187

Some drugs associated with
drug induced lupus:
hydralazine   procainamide
dilantin   isoniazid
less common:
methyldopa   quinidine
sulfonamides   barbiturates
thiouracil   bleomycin
acebutolol   asparaginase
cephalosporins   iodides

SLE - systemic lupus erythematosus
MCTD - mixed connective tissue disease
RA - rheumatoid arthritis
SCLE - subacute cutaneous lupus erythematosus
CHB - congenital heart block
Sm - Smith antigen
PCNA - proliferative cell nuclear antigen
CREST - Calcinosis
         Raynaud's phenomenon
         Esophageal motility disorder
         Scalodactyly, and
         Telangiectasias
         (scleroderma with limited skin involvement)

12a: Management of Diabetic Ketoacidosis

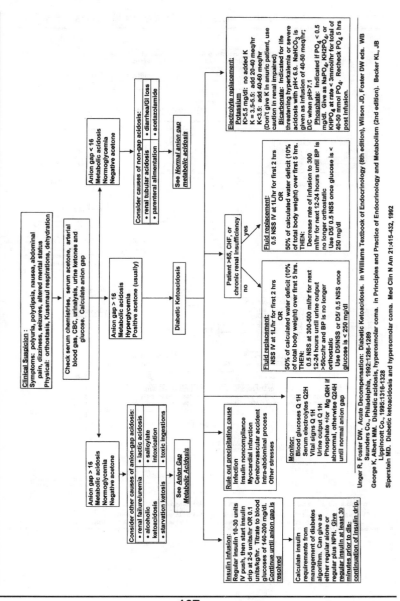

Clinical Suspicion:
Symptoms: polyuria, polydipsia, nausea, abdominal pain, dizziness, seizures, altered mental status
Physical: orthostasis, Kussmaul respirations, dehydration

Check serum chemistries, serum acetone, arterial blood gas, CBC, urinalysis, urine ketones and glucose. Calculate anion gap

Anion gap > 16
Metabolic acidosis
Normoglycemia
Negative acetone

Consider other causes of anion-gap acidosis:
• renal failure/uremia
• alcoholic ketoacidosis
• starvation ketosis
• lactic acidosis
• salicylate intoxication
• toxic ingestions

See Anion Gap Metabolic Acidosis

Insulin Infusion:
Regular insulin 10-30 units IV push, then start insulin drip at 2-5 units/kg/hr OR 0.1 units/kg/hr. Titrate to blood glucoses of 140-200 mg/dl. Continue until anion gap is resolved

Calculate insulin requirements from management of diabetes algorithm. Can give as either regular alone or regular plus NPH. Give regular insulin at least 30 minutes prior to discontinuation of insulin drip.

Rule out precipitating cause
Infection
Insulin noncompliance
Myocardial infarction
Cerebrovascular accident
Intra-abdominal process
Other stresses

Monitor:
Blood glucoses Q 1H
Serum electrolytes Q 2H
Vital signs Q 1H
Urine output Q 1H
Phosphate +/or Mg Q 6H if abnormal, otherwise Q 24H until normal anion gap

Anion gap > 16
Metabolic acidosis
Hyperglycemia
Positive acetone (usually)

Diabetic Ketoacidosis

Patient >65, CHF, or chronic renal insufficiency

no → **Fluid replacement:**
NSS IV at 1L/hr for first 2 hrs
50% of calculated water deficit (10% of total body weight) over first 5 hrs.
THEN:
0.5 NSS at 300-500 ml/hr for next 12-24 hours until urine output >50cc/hr and BP is no longer orthostatic.
Use D5/NSS or D5/ 0.5 NSS once glucose is < 250 mg/dl

yes → **Fluid replacement:**
0.5 NSS IV at 1L/hr for first 2 hrs
50% of calculated water deficit (10% of total body weight) over first 5 hrs.
THEN:
Decrease rate of infusion to 300 ml/hr for next 12-24 hours until BP is no longer orthostatic
Use D5/ 0.5 NSS once glucose is < 250 mg/dl

Anion gap < 16
Metabolic acidosis
Normoglycemia
Negative acetone

Consider causes of non-gap acidosis:
• renal tubular acidosis
• parenteral alimentation
• diarrhea/GI loss
• acetazolamide

See Normal anion gap metabolic acidosis

Electrolyte replacement:
Potassium
K>5.5 mg/dl: no added K
K = 3.5-5.5: add 20-40 meq/hr
K<3.5: add 40-60 meq/hr
(Don't give K in anuric patient, use caution in renal impaired)
Bicarbonate: Indicated for life threatening hyperkalemia or severe acidosis with pH< 6.9. NaHCO$_3$ is given as infusion of 40-50 meq/hr; D/C when pH>7.1
Phosphate: Indicated if PO$_4$ < 0.5 mg/dl. Give as NaPO$_4$, KH$_2$PO$_4$, or KHPO$_4$ at rate < 3mmol/hr for total of 40-50 mmol PO$_4$. Recheck PO$_4$ 5 hrs post infusion.

Unger R, Foster DW. Acute Decompensation: Diabetic Ketoacidosis. in Williams Textbook of Endocrinology (8th edition), Wilson JD, Foster DW eds. WB Saunders Co., Philadelphia, 1992:1286-1289
George K, Albert MM. Diabetic acidosis, hyperosmolar coma. in Principles and Practice of Endocrinology and Metabolism (2nd edition), Becker KL, JB Lippincott Co., 1995:1316-1328
Siperstein MD. Diabetic ketoacidosis and hypersomolar coma. Med Clin N Am 21:415-432, 1992

12b: Management of Diabetes Mellitus

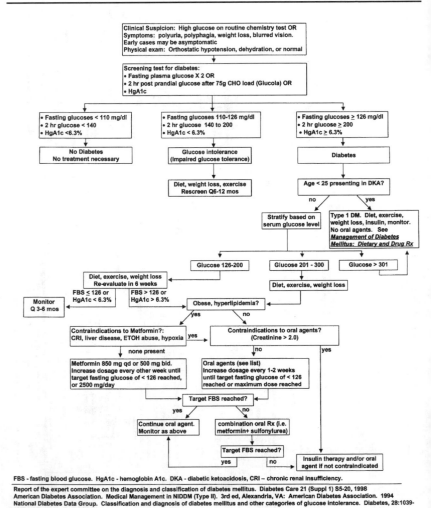

FBS - fasting blood glucose. HgA1c - hemoglobin A1c. DKA - diabetic ketoacidosis, CRI – chronic renal insufficiency.

Report of the expert committee on the diagnosis and classification of diabetes mellitus. Diabetes Care 21 (Suppl 1) S5-20, 1998
American Diabetes Association. Medical Management in NIDDM (Type II). 3rd ed, Alexandria, VA: American Diabetes Association. 1994
National Diabetes Data Group. Classification and diagnosis of diabetes mellitus and other categories of glucose intolerance. Diabetes, 28:1039-1057, 1979
Gerich JE. Oral hypoglycemic agents. N Engl J Med 321:1231-1245, 1989

12c: Management of Diabetes Mellitus: Dietary and Drug Therapy

<u>Diet:</u> ADA (60% CHO, 20% PRO, 20% FAT); add HS snack if on oral hypoglycemic. Add 3 pm + HS snacks if pt on intermediate or long acting insulin (NPH, Lente, Ultralente)

<u>Insulin therapy:</u>
Types of insulin:
1. Short acting: Regular, Humalog
2. Intermediate acting: NPH, Lente
3. Long acting: Ultra Lente

- Starting dose = 0.5-1.0 units/kg/day
- 2/3 given 30' before breakfast: 1/3 short acting, 2/3 intermediate or long acting
- 1/3 given 30' before supper: 1/3 short acting, 2/3 intermediate or long acting
- Insulin must be further adjusted based on patient home monitored blood glucose.

Target blood glucoses:
- AC 80 – 120
- HS 100 – 140
- HgbA1c < 7%

Sulfonylurea	Initial dose	Maximum dose	Contraindications
Glipizide (Glucotrol)	2.5 - 5 mg QD	40 mg po in divided doses	Renal insufficiency (creatinine > 2.0)
Glipizide long acting (Glucotrol XL)	5 mg QD	20 mg daily	
Glyburide (Diabeta, Micronase)	1.25 mg QD	20 mg in divided doses	
Glimepiride (Amaryl)	1-2 mg qd	8 mg qd	
Micronized glyburide (Glynase PT)	1.5 – 3.0 mg qd	12 mg qd	
Other agents	initial dose	maximum dose	Contraindications
Metformin (Glucophage)	500 mg bid	2,500 mg in divided doses	Renal insufficiency, ↑ LFTs, hypoxia, ETOH abuse
Troglitazone (Rezulin)	200 mg qd	600 mg qd	↑ LFTs, ETOH abuse
Acarbose (Precose)	25 mg tid with meals	100 mg tid with meals	↑ LFTs
Repaglinide (Prandin)	0.5 mg tid – qid before meals	4 mg po tid – qid before meals	Renal insufficiency

Possible combinations of oral agents:
1. Sulfonylurea + metformin
2. Sulfonylurea + troglitazone
3. Sulfonylurea + acarbose
4. Metformin + troglitazone
5. Metformin + acarbose
6. Metformin + repaglinide
6. Oral agent plus insulin

<u>Monitoring:</u>
- Initial home glucose monitoring if taking insulin AC and HS
- FBS TIW X 3 weeks for Type 2 diabetes
- HgA1c Q 3 mos
- PE with neurologic exam, peripheral pulses Q 3 mos
- Eye exam (retinopathy) Q 12 mos
- Serum creatinine, 24 hr urine for microalbuminuria + creatinine Q 12 mos
- EKG, stress test for clinical indications

12d: Management of Hypothyroidism

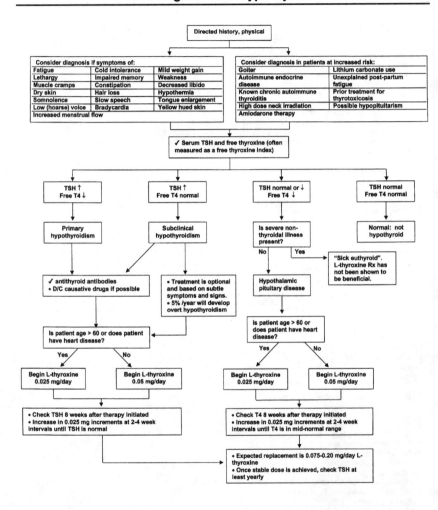

Directed history, physical

Consider diagnosis if symptoms of:

Fatigue	Cold intolerance	Mild weight gain
Lethargy	Impaired memory	Weakness
Muscle cramps	Constipation	Decreased libido
Dry skin	Hair loss	Hypothermia
Somnolence	Slow speech	Tongue enlargement
Low (hoarse) voice	Bradycardia	Yellow hued skin
Increased menstrual flow		

Consider diagnosis in patients at increased risk:

Goiter	Lithium carbonate use
Autoimmune endocrine disease	Unexplained post-partum fatigue
Known chronic autoimmune thyroiditis	Prior treatment for thyrotoxicosis
High dose neck irradiation	Possible hypopituitarism
Amiodarone therapy	

✓ Serum TSH and free thyroxine (often measured as a free thyroxine index)

TSH ↑ / Free T4 ↓

Primary hypothyroidism

- ✓ antithyroid antibodies
- D/C causative drugs if possible

Is patient age > 60 or does patient have heart disease?

Yes → Begin L-thyroxine 0.025 mg/day

No → Begin L-thyroxine 0.05 mg/day

- Check TSH 8 weeks after therapy initiated
- Increase in 0.025 mg increments at 2-4 week intervals until TSH is normal

TSH ↑ / Free T4 normal

Subclinical hypothyroidism

- Treatment is optional and based on subtle symptoms and signs.
- 5% /year will develop overt hypothyroidism

TSH normal or ↓ / Free T4 ↓

Is severe non-thyroidal illness present?

No → Hypothalamic pituitary disease

Yes → "Sick euthyroid". L-thyroxine Rx has not been shown to be beneficial.

Is patient age > 60 or does patient have heart disease?

Yes → Begin L-thyroxine 0.025 mg/day

No → Begin L-thyroxine 0.05 mg/day

- Check T4 8 weeks after therapy initiated
- Increase in 0.025 mg increments at 2-4 week intervals until T4 is in mid-normal range

TSH normal / Free T4 normal

Normal: not hypothyroid

- Expected replacement is 0.075-0.20 mg/day L-thyroxine
- Once stable dose is achieved, check TSH at least yearly

12e: Management of Thyrotoxicosis

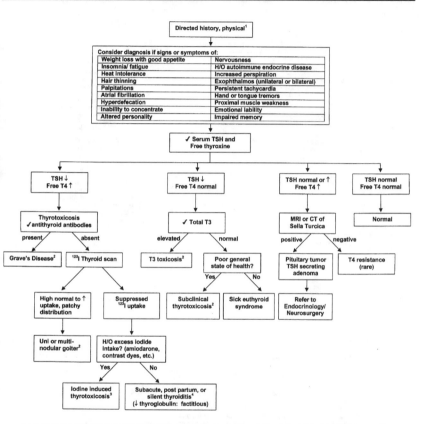

1. Grave's disease goiters are generally smooth. Multinodular goiters have nodules of different sizes. Uninodular glands have a solitary nodule which may consume much of a lobe. Subacute thyroiditis often presents with viral prodrome, persistent neck tenderness and sore throat. The ESR is increased. Post partum thyroiditis may present with thyrotoxicosis or hypothyroidism.

2. Treat with propylthiouracil (PTU, start at 100 mg TID) or methimazole (start at 10-30 mg QD) until T4 levels depleted (1 to several months). β-blockers for symptomatic relief. Refer to Endocrinology for ^{131}I ablation (contraindicated in pregnancy; many avoid use of ^{131}I in children and fertile women; higher doses required for nodular goiter). Surgical excision is an option for Graves' disease and resistant nodules. Monitor for hypothyroidism after treatment.

3. Treat with PTU or methimazole plus β-blockers until thyroidal iodine is depleted. If amiodarone is required, antithyroid drugs can be continued.

4. Usually self limited. β-blockers useful for symptomatic relief of thyrotoxicosis. ASA for neck tenderness. For severe thyrotoxicosis or pain, may use prednisone 40-60 mg/day, taper over 7-10 days. Selected patients benefit from continued prednisone 10 mg/d until normal ^{125}I uptake is restored.

Note: In severe recalcitrant thyrotoxicosis in the medically unstable patient, high dose PTU (600-1000mg/d), ipodate sodium (0.5 g/d), and prednisone 60 mg/d can be given until surgical resection of the thyroid can be safely undertaken

12f: Adrenal Insufficiency

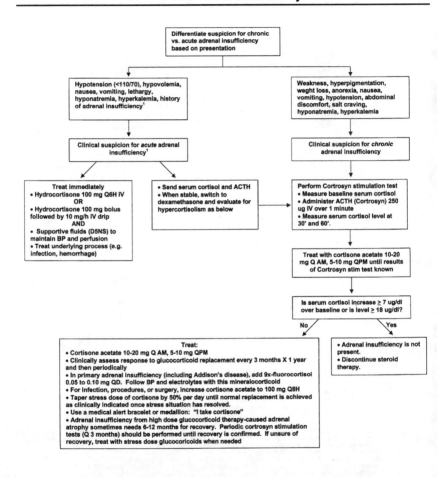

Differentiate suspicion for chronic vs. acute adrenal insufficiency based on presentation

↓

Left branch:

Hypotension (<110/70), hypovolemia, nausea, vomiting, lethargy, hyponatremia, hyperkalemia, history of adrenal insufficiency[1]

↓

Clinical suspicion for *acute* adrenal insufficiency[1]

Treat immediately
- Hydrocortisone 100 mg Q6H IV
  OR
- Hydrocortisone 100 mg bolus followed by 10 mg/h IV drip
  AND
- Supportive fluids (D5NS) to maintain BP and perfusion
- Treat underlying process (e.g. infection, hemorrhage)

- Send serum cortisol and ACTH
- When stable, switch to dexamethasone and evaluate for hypercortisolism as below

Right branch:

Weakness, hyperpigmentation, weight loss, anorexia, nausea, vomiting, hypotension, abdominal discomfort, salt craving, hyponatremia, hyperkalemia

↓

Clinical suspicion for *chronic* adrenal insufficiency

↓

Perform Cortrosyn stimulation test
- Measure baseline serum cortisol
- Administer ACTH (Cortrosyn) 250 ug IV over 1 minute
- Measure serum cortisol level at 30' and 60'.

↓

Treat with cortisone acetate 10-20 mg Q AM, 5-10 mg QPM until results of Cortrosyn stim test known

↓

Is serum cortisol increase ≥ 7 ug/dl over baseline or is level ≥ 18 ug/dl?

No → **Treat:**
- Cortisone acetate 10-20 mg Q AM, 5-10 mg QPM
- Clinically assess response to glucocorticoid replacement every 3 months X 1 year and then periodically
- In primary adrenal insufficiency (including Addison's disease), add 9x-fluorocortisol 0.05 to 0.10 mg QD. Follow BP and electrolytes with this mineralocorticoid
- For infection, procedures, or surgery, increase cortisone acetate to 100 mg Q8H
- Taper stress dose of cortisone by 50% per day until normal replacement is achieved as clinically indicated once stress situation has resolved.
- Use a medical alert bracelet or medallion: "I take cortisone"
- Adrenal insufficiency from high dose glucocorticoid therapy-caused adrenal atrophy sometimes needs 6-12 months for recovery. Periodic cortrosyn stimulation tests (Q 3 months) should be performed until recovery is confirmed. If unsure of recovery, treat with stress dose glucocoricoids when needed

Yes →
- Adrenal insufficiency is not present.
- Discontinue steroid therapy.

1. In acute setting (sepsis, hemorrhage), hyperpigmentation probably will not accompany metabolic effects of hypoadrenalism. In sudden glucocorticoid withdrawal in patients on chronic glucocorticoid therapy, aldosterone is intact and K+ is normal.

12g: Cushing's Syndrome

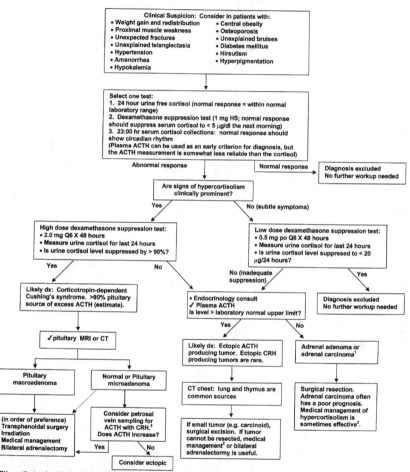

Clinical Suspicion: Consider in patients with:
- Weight gain and redistribution
- Proximal muscle weakness
- Unexpected fractures
- Unexplained telangiectasia
- Hypertension
- Amenorrhea
- Hypokalemia
- Central obesity
- Osteoporosis
- Unexplained bruises
- Diabetes mellitus
- Hirsutism
- Hyperpigmentation

Select one test:
1. 24 hour urine free cortisol (normal response = within normal laboratory range)
2. Dexamethasone suppression test (1 mg HS; normal response should suppress serum cortisol to < 5 μg/dl the next morning)
3. 23:00 hr serum cortisol collections: normal response should show circadian rhythm
(Plasma ACTH can be used as an early criterion for diagnosis, but the ACTH measurement is somewhat less reliable than the cortisol)

Abnormal response → Are signs of hypercortisolism clinically prominent?

Normal response → Diagnosis excluded. No further workup needed

Yes → High dose dexamethasone suppression test:
- 2.0 mg Q6 X 48 hours
- Measure urine cortisol for last 24 hours
- Is urine cortisol level suppressed by > 90%?

No (subtle symptoms) → Low dose dexamethasone suppression test:
- 0.5 mg po Q6 X 48 hours
- Measure urine cortisol for last 24 hours
- Is urine cortisol level suppresed to < 20 μg/24 hours?

Yes → Likely dx: Corticotropin-dependent Cushing's syndrome. >90% pituitary source of excess ACTH (estimate).

No →

No (inadequate suppression) → • Endocrinology consult ✓ Plasma ACTH. Is level > laboratory normal upper limit?

Yes → Diagnosis excluded. No further workup needed

✓ pituitary MRI or CT

Pituitary macroadenoma

Normal or Pituitary microadenoma

Yes → Likely dx: Ectopic ACTH producing tumor. Ectopic CRH producing tumors are rare.

No → Adrenal adenoma or adrenal carcinoma[1]

(in order of preference)
Transphenoidal surgery
Irradiation
Medical management
Bilateral adrenalectomy

Consider petrosal vein sampling for ACTH with CRH.[3] Does ACTH increase?
Yes / No

Consider ectopic

CT chest: lung and thymus are common sources

Surgical resection. Adrenal carcinoma often has a poor prognosis. Medical management of hypercortisolism is sometimes effective[2].

If small tumor (e.g. carcinoid), surgical excision. If tumor cannot be resected, medical management[2] or bilateral adrenalectomy is useful.

CRH – corticotropin releasing hormone. May attain greater usefulness as screening test in the future. About 65% of patients with Cushing's syndrome have a pituitary source for ↑ ACTH (Cushing's disease). Rapid onset of Cushing's syndrome with hyperpigmentation and hypokalemia increase probability of ectopic ACTH source. No test for diagnosing Cushing's is absolute.
1. Adrenal adenomas are mainly cortisol producers with little or no androgens. Adrenal carcinomas are often > 5 cm and may produce a variety of hormones including adrenal androgens or may be silent.
2. Ketoconazole 600-1200 mg/d is drug of choice but has liver toxicity. Metyrapone with aminoglutethimide or mitotane is also useful. Patients with ectopic ACTH tumors can break through medical therapy.
3. Controversial. A non-pituitary source would be rare and petrosal vein sampling is not always available. Dashed line indicates acceptable alernative

13a: Diagnosis and Treatment of Primary Headache

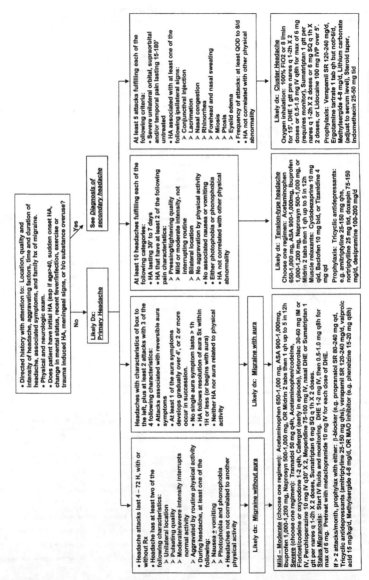

- Directed history with attention to: Location, quality and intensity of headache, aggravating factors, time and duration of headache, associated symptoms, and family fx of migraine.
- Physical and neurologic exam.
- Does patient have initial HA (esp if age>40, sudden onset HA, change in mental status, recent fever/infection, exercise or trauma induced HA, meningeal signs, or h/o substance overuse?

Yes → See Diagnosis of secondary headache

No → Likely Dx: Primary Headache

Migraine without aura

- Headache attacks last 4 – 72 H, with or without Rx
- Headache has at least two of the following characteristics:
  - Unilateral location
  - Pulsating quality
  - Moderate/severe intensity interrupts normal activity
  - Aggravated by routine physical activity
- During headache, at least one of the following:
  - Nausea ± vomiting
  - Photophobia and phonophobia
- Headaches not correlated to another physical activity

Likely dx: Migraine without aura

Mild – Moderate (choose one regimen): Acetaminophen 650-1,000 mg, ASA 900-1,000mg, Ibuprofen 1,000-1,200 mg, Naprosyn 500-1,000 mg, OR Midrin 2 tabs then 1 qh up to 5 in 12h Severe (choose one regimen): Tramadol 50 mg q4h, Acetaminophen/codeine, Florice/codeine or oxycodone 1-2 q4h, Cafergot (early in episode), Ketorolac 30-60 mg IM or IV, Perchlorperazine 10 mg IV q30' X 2, Meperidine 75-100 mg IV, nasal DHE or Sumatriptan 1 gtt per nares q 1-2h X 2 doses, Sumatriptan 6 mg SQ q 1h X 2 doses. Status Migrainosis: Start IV fluids and monitoring. DHE 1-2 mg IV, then 0.5-1.0 mg q8h for max of 6 mg. Pretreat with metaclopramide 10 mg IV for each dose of DHE.

If > 2 attacks/month, prophylax with either: β-blocker (e.g. propranolol SR 80-240 mg qd, Tricyclic antidepressants (amitriptyline 25-150 mg qhs), verapamil SR 120-240 mg qd, valproic acid 15 mg/kg/d, Methylsergide 4-8 mg/d, OR MAO inhibitor (e.g. phenelzine 15-20 mg q8h)

Migraine with aura

- Headaches with characteristics of box to the left, plus at least 2 attacks with 3 of the 4 following characteristics:
  - Attacks associated with reversible aura symptoms
  - At least 1 of the aura symptoms develops gradually over 4', or 2 or more occur in succession.
  - No single aura symptom lasts > 1h
  - HA follows resolution of aura Sx within 1H or less (or begins with aura)
  - Neither HA nor aura related to physical activity

Likely dx: Migraine with aura

Tension-type headache

- At least 10 headaches fulfilling each of the following categories:
  - HA lasting 30 to 7 days
  - HA that have at least 2 of the following pain characteristics:
    - Pressing/tightening quality
    - Mild or moderate intensity, not interrupting routine
    - Bilateral location
    - No aggravation by physical activity
  - No associated nausea or vomiting
  - Either photophobia or phonophobia
  - HA not correlated with other physical abnormality

Likely dx: Tension-type headache

Choose one regimen: Acetaminophen 650-1,000 mg, ASA 900-1,000mg, Ibuprofen 1,000-1,200 mg, Naprosyn 500-1,000 mg, or Midrin 2 tabs then 1 qh up to 5 in 12h Muscle relaxants: Cyclobenzaprine 10 mg qid, Baclofen 10 mg bid, or Tizanidine 4 mg qd

Prophylaxis: Tricyclic antidepressants: e.g. amitriptyline 25-150 mg qhs, nortriptyline 25 mg tid, doxepin 75-150 mg/d, desipramine 100-200 mg/d

Cluster Headache

- At least 5 attacks fulfilling each of the following criteria:
  - Severe unilateral orbital, supraorbital and/or temporal pain lasting 15-180' untreated
  - HA associated with at least one of the following ipsilateral signs:
    - Conjunctival Injection
    - Lacrimation
    - Nasal congestion
    - Rhinorrhea
    - Forehead and nasal sweating
    - Miosis
    - Ptosis
    - Eyelid edema
  - Frequency of attacks: at least QOD to 8/d
  - HA not correlated with other physical abnormality

Likely dx: Cluster Headache

Oxygen inhalation: 100% FIO2 or 8 l/min for 15', DHE 1 gtt pre nares q 1-2h X 2 doses or 0.5-1.0 mg IV q8h for max of 6 mg (requires monitor), Sumatriptan 1 gtt per nares q 1-2h X 2 doses or 6 mg SQ 1h X 2 doses, or Lidocaine 100 mg IVP over 5'.

Prophylaxis: Verapamil SR 120-240 mg/d, Ergotamine tartrate 1 tab qh but nob>6/d, Methylsergide 4-8 mg/d, Lithium carbonate (adjust to serum level), Steroid taper, Indomethacin 25-50 mg tid

Cuter M. Headache in Borsook D, LeBel AA, McPeak B (eds). The Massachussetts General Hospital Handbook of Pain Management. Little Brown, Boston, 1995: 270-302

13b: Diagnosis of Secondary Headache

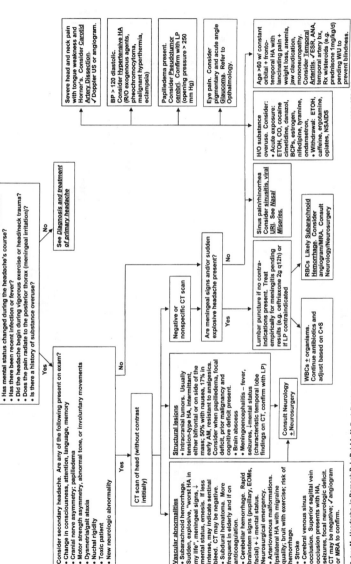

Cutrer M. Headache. in Borsook D, LeBel AA, McPeak B (eds). The Massachussetts General Hospital Handbook of Pain Management. Little Brown, Boston; 1995: 270-302

13c: Coma and Drowsiness

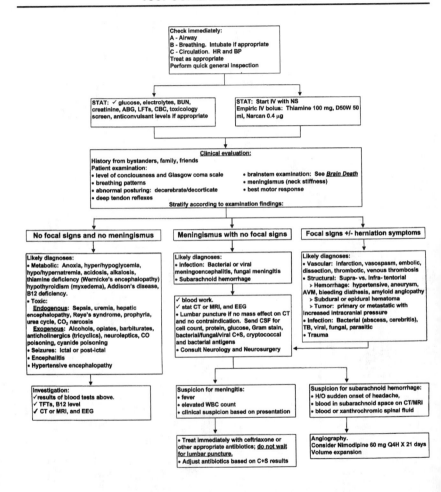

Check immediately:
A - Airway
B - Breathing. Intubate if appropriate
C - Circulation. HR and BP
Treat as appropriate
Perform quick general inspection

STAT: ✓ glucose, electrolytes, BUN, creatinine, ABG, LFTs, CBC, toxicology screen, anticonvulsant levels if appropriate

STAT: Start IV with NS
Empiric IV bolus: Thiamine 100 mg, D50W 50 ml, Narcan 0.4 μg

Clinical evaluation:
History from bystanders, family, friends
Patient examination:
• level of conciousness and Glasgow coma scale
• breathing patterns
• abnormal posturing: decerebrate/decorticate
• deep tendon reflexes
• brainstem examination: See *Brain Death*
• meningismus (neck stiffness)
• best motor response
Stratify according to examination findings:

No focal signs and no meningismus

Likely diagnoses:
• Metabolic: Anoxia, hyper/hypoglycemia, hypo/hypernatremia, acidosis, alkalosis, thiamine deficiency (Wernicke's encephalopathy) hypothyroidism (myxedema), Addison's disease, B12 deficiency.
• Toxic:
   Endogenous: Sepsis, uremia, hepatic encephalopathy, Reye's syndrome, prophyria, urea cycle, CO_2 narcosis
   Exogenous: Alcohols, opiates, barbiturates, anticholinergics (tricyclics), neuroleptics, CO poisoning, cyanide poisoning
• Seizures: Ictal or post-ictal
• Encephalitis
• Hypertensive encephalopathy

Investigation:
✓ results of blood tests above.
✓ TFTs, B12 level
✓ CT or MRI, and EEG

Meningismus with no focal signs

Likely diagnoses:
• Infection: Bacterial or viral meningoencephalitis, fungal meningitis
• Subarachnoid hemorrhage

✓ blood work.
✓ stat CT or MRI, and EEG
• Lumbar puncture if no mass effect on CT and no contraindication. Send CSF for cell count, protein, glucose, Gram stain, bacterial/fungal/viral C+S, cryptococcal and bacterial antigens
• Consult Neurology and Neurosurgery

Suspicion for meningitis:
• fever
• elevated WBC count
• clinical suspicion based on presentation

• Treat immediately with ceftriaxone or other appropriate antibiotics; do not wait for lumbar puncture.
• Adjust antibiotics based on C+S results

Focal signs +/- herniation symptoms

Likely diagnoses:
• Vascular: infarction, vasospasm, embolic, dissection, thrombotic, venous thrombosis
• Structural: Supra- vs. infra- tentorial
   > Hemorrhage: hypertensive, aneurysm, AVM, bleeding diathesis, amyloid angiopathy
   > Subdural or epidural hematoma
   > Tumor: primary or metastatic with increased intracranial pressure
• Infection: Bacterial (abscess, cerebritis), TB, viral, fungal, parasitic
• Trauma

Suspicion for subarachnoid hemorrhage:
• H/O sudden onset of headache,
• blood in subarachnoid space on CT/MRI
• blood or xanthrochromic spinal fluid

Angiography.
Consider Nimodipine 60 mg Q4H X 21 days
Volume expansion

13d: Status Epilepticus: Diagnostic Algorithm

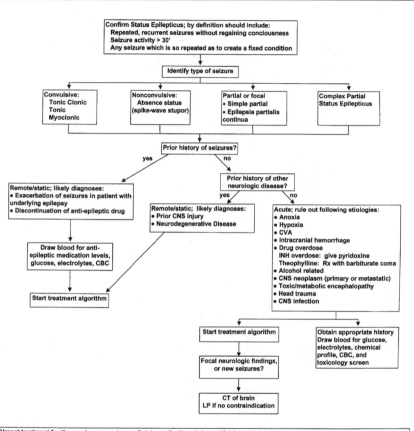

Confirm Status Epilepticus; by definition should include:
Repeated, recurrent seizures without regaining conciousness
Seizure activity > 30'
Any seizure which is so repeated as to create a fixed condition

Identify type of seizure

Convulsive:
Tonic Clonic
Tonic
Myoclonic

Nonconvulsive:
Absence status
(spike-wave stupor)

Partial or focal
• Simple partial
• Epilepsia partialis continua

Complex Partial
Status Epilepticus

Prior history of seizures?

yes   no

Prior history of other neurologic disease?

yes   no

Remote/static; likely diagnoses:
• Exacerbation of seizures in patient with underlying epilepsy
• Discontinuation of anti-epileptic drug

Remote/static; likely diagnoses:
• Prior CNS injury
• Neurodegenerative Disease

Acute; rule out following etiologies:
• Anoxia
• Hypoxia
• CVA
• Intracranial hemorrhage
• Drug overdose
   INH overdose: give pyridoxine
   Theophylline: Rx with barbiturate coma
• Alcohol related
• CNS neoplasm (primary or metastatic)
• Toxic/metabolic encephalopathy
• Head trauma
• CNS infection

Draw blood for anti-epileptic medication levels, glucose, electrolytes, CBC

Start treatment algorithm

Start treatment algorithm

Focal neurologic findings, or new seizures?

Obtain appropriate history
Draw blood for glucose, electrolytes, chemical profile, CBC, and toxicology screen

CT of brain
LP if no contraindication

Urgent treatment for the most common types of status epilepticus is imperative because:
1. Prolonged (>60') seizures may be associated with neuronal injury
2. The medical problems associated with prolonged status can be severe and life threatening
3. Status epilepticus can be seen in association with other neurologic or medical emergencies (i.e. intracerebral hemorrhage, CNS infection).
4. The longer status epilepticus persists, the more refractory it becomes

Sequelae of Status Epilepticus:
Most are preventable with approprate treatment of status epilepticus and associated medical concomitants

Hypoxia	Lactic acidosis	Rhabdomyolysis
Hyperkalemia	Hyperpyrexia	Leukocytosis
CSF pleocytosis	Aspiration pneumonia	Pulmonary edema
Catecholamine release	Hypertension	Altered cerebral autoregulation
Shock (late)		

13e: Status Epilepticus: Treatment Algorithm

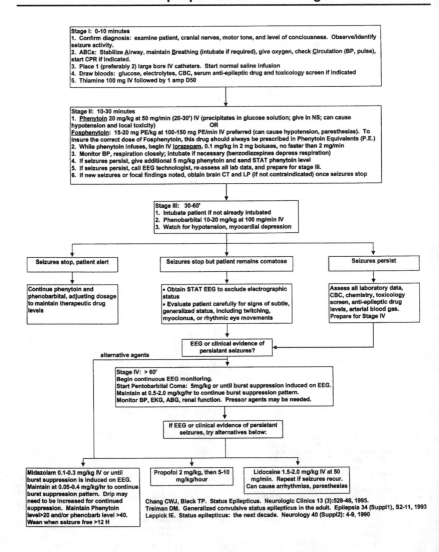

Stage I: 0-10 minutes
1. Confirm diagnosis: examine patient, cranial nerves, motor tone, and level of conciousness. Observe/identify seizure activity.
2. ABCs: Stabilize Airway, maintain Breathing (intubate if required), give oxygen, check Circulation (BP, pulse), start CPR if indicated.
3. Place 1 (preferably 2) large bore IV catheters. Start normal saline infusion
4. Draw bloods: glucose, electrolytes, CBC, serum anti-epileptic drug and toxicology screen if indicated
5. Thiamine 100 mg IV followed by 1 amp D50

Stage II: 10-30 minutes
1. Phenytoin 20 mg/kg at 50 mg/min (20-30') IV (precipitates in glucose solution; give in NS; can cause hypotension and local toxicity) OR
Fosphenytoin: 15-20 mg PE/kg at 100-150 mg PE/min IV preferred (can cause hypotension, paresthesias). To insure the correct dose of Fosphenytoin, this drug should always be prescribed in Phenytoin Equivalents (P.E.)
2. While phenytoin infuses, begin IV lorazepam, 0.1 mg/kg in 2 mg boluses, no faster than 2 mg/min
3. Monitor BP, respiration closely; intubate if necessary (benzodiazepines depress respiration)
4. If seizures persist, give additional 5 mg/kg phenytoin and send STAT phenytoin level
5. If seizures persist, call EEG technologist, re-assess all lab data, and prepare for stage III.
6. If new seizures or focal findings noted, obtain brain CT and LP (if not contraindicated) once seizures stop

Stage III: 30-60'
1. Intubate patient if not already intubated
2. Phenobarbital 10-20 mg/kg at 100 mg/min IV
3. Watch for hypotension, myocardial depression

Seizures stop, patient alert

Continue phenytoin and phenobarbital, adjusting dosage to maintain therapeutic drug levels

Seizures stop but patient remains comatose

- Obtain STAT EEG to exclude electrographic status
- Evaluate patient carefully for signs of subtle, generalized status, including twitching, myoclonus, or rhythmic eye movements

Seizures persist

Assess all laboratory data, CBC, chemistry, toxicology screen, anti-epileptic drug levels, arterial blood gas. Prepare for Stage IV

EEG or clinical evidence of persistant seizures?

alternative agents

Stage IV: > 60'
Begin continuous EEG monitoring.
Start Pentobarbital Coma: 5mg/kg or until burst suppression induced on EEG.
Maintain at 0.5-2.0 mg/kg/hr to continue burst suppression pattern.
Monitor BP, EKG, ABG, renal function. Pressor agents may be needed.

If EEG or clinical evidence of persistant seizures, try alternatives below:

Midazolam 0.1-0.3 mg/kg IV or until burst suppression is induced on EEG. Maintain at 0.05-0.4 mg/kg/hr to continue burst suppression pattern. Drip may need to be increased for continued suppression. Maintain Phenytoin level>20 and/or phenobarb level >40. Wean when seizure free >12 H

Propofol 2 mg/kg, then 5-10 mg/kg/hour

Lidocaine 1.5-2.0 mg/kg IV at 50 mg/min. Repeat if seizures recur. Can cause arrhythmias, paresthesias

Chang CWJ, Bleck TP. Status Epilepticus. Neurologic Clinics 13 (3):529-48, 1995.
Treiman DM. Generalized convulsive status epilepticus in the adult. Epilepsia 34 (Suppl1), S2-11, 1993
Leppick IE. Status epilepticus: the next decade. Neurology 40 (Suppl2): 4-9, 1990

13f: Acute Stroke

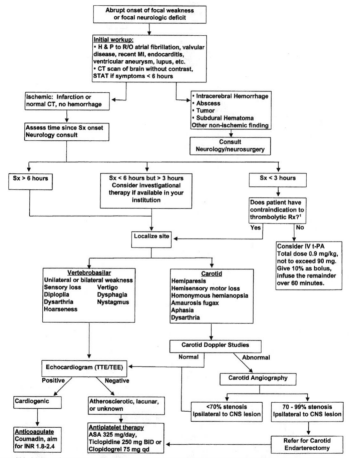

Abrupt onset of focal weakness or focal neurologic deficit

Initial workup:
• H & P to R/O atrial fibrillation, valvular disease, recent MI, endocarditis, ventricular aneurysm, lupus, etc.
• CT scan of brain without contrast, STAT if symptoms < 6 hours

Ischemic: Infarction or normal CT, no hemorrhage

• Intracerebral Hemorrhage
• Abscess
• Tumor
• Subdural Hematoma
Other non-ischemic finding

Assess time since Sx onset
Neurology consult

Consult
Neurology/neurosurgery

Sx > 6 hours

Sx < 6 hours but > 3 hours
Consider investigational therapy if available in your institution

Sx < 3 hours

Does patient have contraindication to thrombolytic Rx?[1]
Yes   No

Consider IV t-PA
Total dose 0.9 mg/kg, not to exceed 90 mg. Give 10% as bolus, infuse the remainder over 60 minutes.

Localize site

Vertebrobasilar
Unilateral or bilateral weakness
Sensory loss   Vertigo
Diploplia   Dysphagia
Dysarthria   Nystagmus
Hoarseness

Carotid
Hemiparesis
Hemisensory motor loss
Homonymous hemianopsia
Amaurosis fugax
Aphasia
Dysarthria

Carotid Doppler Studies
Normal   Abnormal

Echocardiogram (TTE/TEE)
Positive   Negative

Carotid Angiography

Cardiogenic

Atherosclerotic, lacunar, or unknown

<70% stenosis
Ipsilateral to CNS lesion

70 - 99% stenosis
Ipsilateral to CNS lesion

Anticoagulate
Coumadin, aim for INR 1.8-2.4

Antiplatelet therapy
ASA 325 mg/day,
Ticlopidine 250 mg BID or
Clopidogrel 75 mg qd

Refer for Carotid Endarterectomy

[1]CVA or head trauma within 3 mos, major surgery within 14 days, h/o intracranial hemorrhage, BP > 185 systolic or 110 diastolic, rapidly improving or minor Sx, Sx suggestive of subarachnoid hemorrhage, GI or GU hemorrhage within 21 days, arterial puncture at a noncompressible site within 7 days, seizure at onset of stroke.

The National Institute of Neurological Disorders and Stroke rt-PA stroke study group. Tissue Plasminogen Activator for acute ischemic stroke. N Engl J Med 1995, 333:1581-1587

Chanerro A, Vica N, Saiz A, Aidery, Tolosa E. Early anticoagulation of the large cerebral infarction: a safety study. Neurology 1995; 45:861-865

Bellavane A. Efficacy of ticlopidine and aspirin for prevention of reversable cerebrovascular ischemic events: The ticlopidine aspirin stroke study. 1993; 24:1452-1457

13g: Secondary Prevention of Ischemic Stroke

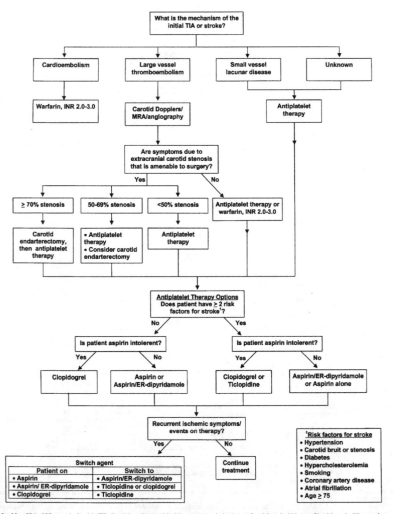

What is the mechanism of the initial TIA or stroke?

- Cardioembolism → Warfarin, INR 2.0-3.0
- Large vessel thromboembolism → Carotid Dopplers/MRA/angiography
- Small vessel lacunar disease → Antiplatelet therapy
- Unknown → Antiplatelet therapy

Are symptoms due to extracranial carotid stenosis that is amenable to surgery?

Yes
- ≥ 70% stenosis → Carotid endarterectomy, then antiplatelet therapy
- 50-69% stenosis → • Antiplatelet therapy • Consider carotid endarterectomy
- <50% stenosis → Antiplatelet therapy

No → Antiplatelet therapy or warfarin, INR 2.0-3.0

Antiplatelet Therapy Options
Does patient have ≥ 2 risk factors for stroke[1]?

No → Is patient aspirin intolerent?
- Yes → Clopidogrel
- No → Aspirin or Aspirin/ER-dipyridamole

Yes → Is patient aspirin intolerent?
- Yes → Clopidogrel or Ticlopidine
- No → Aspirin/ER-dipyridamole or Aspirin alone

Recurrent ischemic symptoms/events on therapy?

No → Continue treatment

Yes → Switch agent

Patient on	Switch to
• Aspirin	• Aspirin/ER-dipyridamole
• Aspirin/ ER-dipyridamole	• Ticlopidine or clopidogrel
• Clopidogrel	• Ticlopidine

[1]Risk factors for stroke
- Hypertension
- Carotid bruit or stenosis
- Diabetes
- Hypercholesterolemia
- Smoking
- Coronary artery disease
- Atrial fibrillation
- Age ≥ 75

Aspirin: 50 to 325 mg qd. Aspirin/ER-pyridamole: aspirin 25 mg + extended release dipyridamole 200 mg. Clopidogrel: 75 mg qd. Ticlopidine: 250 mg bid-

Fayad PB. Ischemic Cerebrovascular Disease. in Rakel RE ed. Conn's Current Therapy 1999. WB Saunders Co., Philadelphia, 885-91, 1999
Albers GW et al. Antithrombotic and Thrombolytic Therapy for Ischemic Stroke. Chest 114: 683S-98S, 1998

13h: Parkinson's Disease

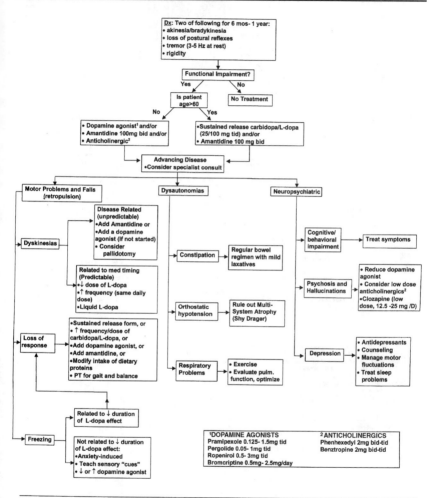

Dx: Two of following for 6 mos- 1 year:
- akinesia/bradykinesia
- loss of postural reflexes
- tremor (3-5 Hz at rest)
- rigidity

Functional Impairment?

Yes → Is patient age>60

No → No Treatment

Is patient age>60:
- No → • Dopamine agonist[1] and/or • Amantidine 100mg bid and/or • Anticholinergic[2]
- Yes → • Sustained release carbidopa/L-dopa (25/100 mg tid) and/or • Amantidine 100 mg bid

Advancing Disease
• Consider specialist consult

Motor Problems and Falls (retropulsion)

Dyskinesias:
- Disease Related (unpredictable)
  - Add Amantidine or
  - Add a dopamine agonist (if not started)
  - Consider pallidotomy
- Related to med timing (Predictable)
  - ↓ dose of L-dopa
  - ↑ frequency (same daily dose)
  - Liquid L-dopa

Loss of response:
- Sustained release form, or
- ↑ frequency/dose of carbidopa/L-dopa, or
- Add dopamine agonist, or
- Add amantidine, or
- Modify intake of dietary proteins
- PT for gait and balance

Freezing:
- Related to ↓ duration of L-dopa effect
- Not related to ↓ duration of L-dopa effect:
  - Anxiety-induced
  - Teach sensory "cues"
  - ↓ or ↑ dopamine agonist

Dysautonomias

Constipation → Regular bowel regimen with mild laxatives

Orthostatic hypotension → Rule out Multi-System Atrophy (Shy Drager)

Respiratory Problems → • Exercise • Evaluate pulm. function, optimize

Neuropsychiatric

Cognitive/behavioral impairment → Treat symptoms

Psychosis and Hallucinations → • Reduce dopamine agonist • Consider low dose anticholinergics[2] • Clozapine (low dose, 12.5 -25 mg /D)

Depression → • Antidepressants • Counseling • Manage motor fluctuations • Treat sleep problems

[1]DOPAMINE AGONISTS
Pramipexole 0.125- 1.5mg tid
Pergolide 0.05- 1mg tid
Ropenirol 0.5- 3mg tid
Bromcriptine 0.5mg- 2.5mg/day

[2] ANTICHOLINERGICS
Phenhexedyl 2mg bid-tid
Benztropine 2mg bid-tid

Kurlan R. 1995.Treatment of Movement Disorders. JB Lippincott, Philadephia

13i: Brain Death

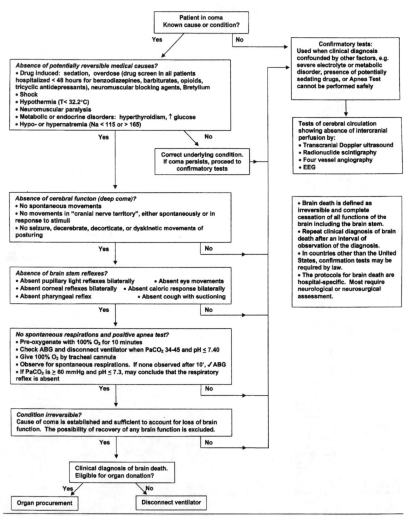

Patient in coma
Known cause or condition?

Yes / No

Absence of potentially reversible medical causes?
• Drug induced: sedation, overdose (drug screen in all patients hospitalized < 48 hours for benzodiazepines, barbiturates, opioids, tricyclic antidepressants), neuromuscular blocking agents, Bretylium
• Shock
• Hypothermia (T< 32.2°C)
• Neuromuscular paralysis
• Metabolic or endocrine disorders: hyperthyroidism, ↑ glucose
• Hypo- or hypernatremia (Na < 115 or > 165)

Yes / No

Correct underlying condition.
If coma persists, proceed to confirmatory tests

Absence of cerebral function (deep coma)?
• No spontaneous movements
• No movements in "cranial nerve territory", either spontaneously or in response to stimuli
• No seizure, decerebrate, decorticate, or dyskinetic movements of posturing

Yes / No

Absence of brain stem reflexes?
• Absent pupillary light reflexes bilaterally   • Absent eye movements
• Absent corneal reflexes bilaterally   • Absent caloric response bilaterally
• Absent pharyngeal reflex   • Absent cough with suctioning

Yes / No

No spontaneous respirations and positive apnea test?
• Pre-oxygenate with 100% O_2 for 10 minutes
• Check ABG and disconnect ventilator when $PaCO_2$ 34-45 and pH ≤ 7.40
• Give 100% O_2 by tracheal cannula
• Observe for spontaneous respirations. If none observed after 10', ✓ ABG
• If $PaCO_2$ is ≥ 60 mmHg and pH ≤ 7.3, may conclude that the respiratory reflex is absent

Yes / No

Condition irreversible?
Cause of coma is established and sufficient to account for loss of brain function. The possibility of recovery of any brain function is excluded.

Yes / No

Clinical diagnosis of brain death.
Eligible for organ donation?

Yes / No

Organ procurement / **Disconnect ventilator**

Confirmatory tests:
Used when clinical diagnosis confounded by other factors, e.g. severe electrolyte or metabolic disorder, presence of potentially sedating drugs, or Apnea Test cannot be performed safely

Tests of cerebral circulation showing absence of intercranial perfusion by:
• Transcranial Doppler ultrasound
• Radionuclide scintigraphy
• Four vessel angiography
• EEG

• Brain death is defined as irreversible and complete cessation of all functions of the brain including the brain stem.
• Repeat clinical diagnosis of brain death after an interval of observation of the diagnosis.
• In countries other than the United States, confirmation tests may be required by law.
• The protocols for brain death are hospital-specific. Most require neurological or neurosurgical assessment.

Halevy A and Brody B. Brain death: Reconciling definitions, criteria, and tests. Ann Intern Med 119: 519-525, 1993
President's commission for the study of ethical problems in medicine and biomedical and behavioral research. Defining death: a report on the medical, legal, and ethical issues in the determination of death. Washington, DC. The Commission, 1981

14a: Initial Management of Oral Overdoses

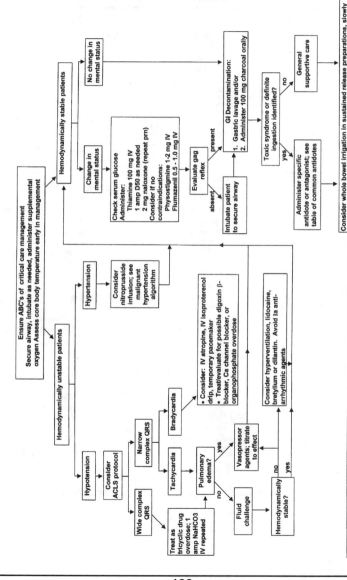

Ensure ABC's of critical care management
Secure airway, intubate as needed, administer supplemental oxygen. Assess core body temperature early in management

Hemodynamically unstable patients

Hypotension — Consider ACLS protocol

Wide complex QRS → Treat as tricyclic drug overdose; 1 amp NaHCO3 IV repeated

Narrow complex QRS

Tachycardia

Bradycardia

• Consider: IV atropine, IV isoproterenol drip, temporary pacemaker
• Treat/evaluate for possible digoxin β-blocker, Ca channel blocker, or organophosphate overdose

Pulmonary edema?
yes → Vasopressor agents; titrate to effect
no → Fluid challenge

Hemodynamically stable?
no
yes

Consider hyperventilation, lidocaine, bretylium or dilantin. Avoid Ia anti-arrhythmic agents

Hypertension — Consider nitroprusside infusion; see malignant hypertension algorithm

Hemodynamically stable patients

Change in mental status

No change in mental status

Check serum glucose
Administer:
Thiamine 100 mg IV
1 amp D50 as needed
2 mg naloxone (repeat prn)
Consider if no contraindications:
Physostigmine 1-2 mg IV
Flumazenil 0.5 - 1.0 mg IV

Evaluate gag reflex
present
absent → Intubate patient to secure airway

GI Decontamination:
1. Gastric lavage and/or
2. Administer 100 mg charcoal orally

Toxic syndrome or definite ingestion identified?
yes → Administer specific antidote or antagonist; see table of common antidotes
no → General supportive care

Consider whole bowel irrigation in sustained release preparations, slowly dissolving agents (iron, button batteries), ingested drug containing packets (use polyethylene glycol 1-2L/hr in adults, 0.5L/hr in children until rectal effluent is clear)
Consider multiple dose charcoal for the first 24 hours (0.5-1 gm/kg q6hr)

Kulig K. Initial management of ingestions of toxic substances. N Eng l J Med , 326(25);1677-1681, 1992.
Flomenbaum NE, et al. General management of the poisoned or overdosed patient. In Goldfrank LR et al (eds) *Goldfrank's Toxicologic Emergencies, 5th ed,* Appleton & Lange, Norwalk, 1994, p 25-42

Acetaminophen	N-acetylcysteine: 140 mg/kg oral loading dose, 70 mg/kg po q4h x 17 doses
Anticholinergic agents	Physostigmine: 1-2 mg IV over 5 minutes, repeat as needed
Benzodiazepines	Flumazenil: 0.2-0.5 mg IV over 1minute Repeat until effect or up to 5 mg
Beta-blockers	Glucagon: 5-10 mg IV titrate to response Maintenance dose of 2-10 mg may be needed
Calcium channel blockers	Calcium chloride: 1 gm IV over 5 minutes May be repeated often in life-threatening cases Monitor calcium levels
Coumadin	Vitamin K1: 1.5-10mg IV(at 1mg/mn), IM, SQ q4-8h, May repeat in 4-8 hrs per PT times.
Cyanide	Eli Lily Kit Amyl nitrite ampules broken and inhaled Sodium nitrite 10cc of 3% solution IV over 5 minutes Sodium thiosulfate 50cc of 25% solution IV over 10 minutes
Digitalis	Digibind :if unknown amount, begin with 10 vials If known amount, give as number of vials = (mg of digoxin ingested divided by 0.6) If steady state serum level known, number of vials = [concentration (ng/ml) x 5.6 x weight (kg)] divided by 600
Ethylene glycol	Ethanol: 10cc of 10% solution/kg IV loading dose, 0.15cc/kg/hr maintenance dose (see **_Management of Unknown Alcohol Ingestion_**)
Isoniazid	Pyridoxine: If unknown amount, give 5 mg IV + titrate upward If known, equivalent amounts i.e. give mg per mg ingested
Methanol	see ethylene glycol and **_Management of Unknown Alcohol Ingestion_**
Opiates	Naloxone: 0.4-2.0 mg IV initially Titrate upward until effect or until 10 mg is reached without effect
Organophosphates	Atropine: 2 mg IV, titrate upward to dry secretions, may require large doses Pralidoxime:25-50 mg/kg over 5 minutes, may require repeat dosing within 6 H
Tricyclic antidepressants	Sodium bicarbonate: 1-2 mmol/kg IV for cardiac dysrhythmia, repeat as needed

KuligK. Initial management of ingestions of toxic substances. N Engl J Med, 326(25);1677-1681, 1992.

14c: Management of Unknown Alcohol Ingestion

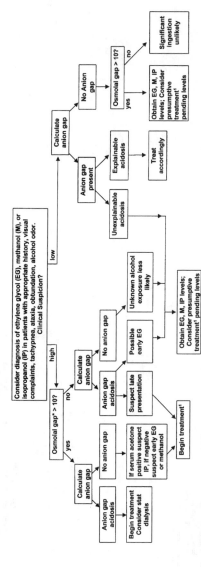

Consider diagnosis of ethylene glycol (EG), methanol (M), or isopropanol (IP) in patients with appropriate history, visual complaints, tachypnea, ataxia, obtundation, alcohol odor. Clinical Suspicion?

high

Osmolal gap* > 10?

— yes → Calculate anion gap
- No anion gap → If serum acetone positive suspect IP, if negative suspect early EG or methanol
- Anion gap acidosis → Begin treatment. Consider stat dialysis

— no → Calculate anion gap
- Anion gap acidosis → Suspect late presentation → Begin treatment[1]
- No anion gap → Possible early EG → Obtain EG, M, IP levels; Consider presumptive treatment[1] pending levels
- Unknown alcohol exposure less likely

low

Calculate anion gap
- Anion gap present
  - Unexplainable acidosis → Obtain EG, M, IP levels; Consider presumptive treatment[1] pending levels
  - Explainable acidosis → Treat accordingly
- No Anion gap → Osmolal gap > 10?
  - yes → Obtain EG, M, IP levels; Consider presumptive treatment[1] pending levels
  - no → Significant ingestion unlikely

*Osmolal gap = serum measured osmolality - calculated osmolarity [2Na+(BUN/2.8)+(glucose/18)] > 10 mosm = abnormal alcohols, acetone, beta-hydroxy-butyrate, acetoacetate, lactate, mannitol, hyperlipidemia, hyperprothrobinemia will all elevate osmolal gap AG acidosis = anion gap acidosis

1. Treatment = obtain stat EG, M, IP levels
   Administer fomepizole (Antizol) 15 mg/kg bolus, then 10 mg/kg q12h X 4 doses, each infusion over 30 minutes.
   If fomepizole not available, then begin ethanol therapy (assume 0 level at start, maintain at 100-150 mg/dl):
   If not fluid overloaded
       10cc of 10% ethanol per kg, maintenance of 0.15 cc per kg per hr
       in 70 kg person using 10% ethanol solution, load intravenously with 700 cc over 1-2 hours, maintain at 100 cc/hr
       double volume if using 5 % ethanol solution
   if fluid overloaded
       in 70 kg person using 80 proof load with 175 cc orally, maintain at 30 cc/hr
   administer thiamine, pyridoxine, folate
   check ethanol and glucose levels frequently

Glasser DS. Utility of the serum osmol gap in the diagnosis of methanol or ethylene glycol ingestion. Ann Emerg Med; 27(3)343-346
Howland MA, Quattrocchi E. Commonly used infusion rates In Roberts JR, Hedges JR (eds) *Clinical Procedures in Emergency Medicine,* 2nd ed. WB Saunders, Philadelphia, 1991, p 1126-1127.

15a: Urinary Tract Infections

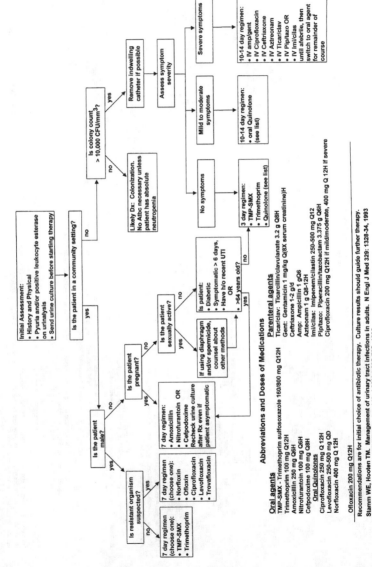

Initial Assessment:
- History and Physical
- Pyuria and/or positive leukocyte esterase on urinalysis
- Send urine culture before starting therapy

Is the patient in a community setting? → no

Is colony count > 10,000 CFU/mm³?
- yes → Remove indwelling catheter if possible → Assess symptom severity
- no → Likely Dx: Colonization. No Atbc necessary unless patient has absolute neutropenia

Assess symptom severity:
- Severe symptoms → **10-14 day regimen:**
  - IV amp/gent
  - IV Ciprofloxacin
  - IV Ceftriaxone
  - IV Aztreonam
  - IV Ticar/clav
  - IV Pip/tazo OR
  - IV Imi/cilas until afebrile, then switch to oral agent for remainder of course
- Mild to moderate symptoms → **10-14 day regimen:**
  - oral Quinolone (see list)
- No symptoms → **3 day regimen:**
  - TMP-SMX
  - Trimethoprim
  - Quinolone (see list)

Is the patient in a community setting? → yes

Is the patient male?
- yes → Is resistant organism suspected?
  - no → **7 day regimen (choose one):**
    - TMP-SMX
    - Trimethoprim
  - yes → **7 day regimen (choose one):**
    - Norfloxin
    - Ofloxin
    - Ciprofloxacin
    - Levofloxacin
    - Trovafloxacin
- no → **Is the patient pregnant?**
  - yes → **7 day regimen:**
    - Amoxicillin
    - Nitrofurantoin OR
    - Cefpodoxime
    Recheck urine culture after Rx even if patient asymptomatic
  - no → **Is the patient sexually active?**
    - yes → If using diaphragm and/or spermicide, counsel about other methods
    - no → **Is patient:**
      - Diabetic
      - Symptomatic > 6 days,
      - Have h/o recent UTI
      OR
      - >64 years old?
        - yes → (7 day regimen)
        - no → **3 day regimen:**
          - TMP-SMX
          - Trimethoprim
          - Quinolone (see list)

Abbreviations and Doses of Medications

Oral agents
TMP-SMX - Trimethoprim sulfosoxazole 160/800 mg Q12H
Trimethoprim 100 mg Q12H
Amoxicillin 250 mg Q8H
Nitrofurantoin 100 mg Q6H
Cefpodoxime 100 mg Q8H

Oral Quinolones
Ciprofloxacin 250 mg Q 12H
Levofloxacin 250-500 mg QD
Norfloxacin 400 mg Q 12H

Ofloxacin 200 mg Q12H

Parenteral agents
Ticar/clav: Ticarcillin/clavulanate 3.2 g Q8H
Gent: Gentamicin 1 mg/kg Q(8X serum creatinine)H
Ceftriaxone 1-2 g/d
Amp: Ampicillin 1 gQ6
Aztreonam 1 g Q6-12H
Imi/cilas: Imipenem/cilastin 250-500 mg Q12
Pip/tazo: Piperacillin/tazobactam 3.375 g Q6H
Ciprofloxacin 200 mg Q12H if mild/moderate, 400 mg Q 12H if severe

---

Recommendations are for initial choice of antibiotic therapy. Culture results should guide further therapy.
Stamm WE, Hooten TM. Management of urinary tract infections in adults. N Engl J Med 329: 1328-34, 1993
Neu HC. Urinary tract infections. Am J Med 92(4a):63S-70S, 1992
Wilkie ME, Almond MK, Marsh FP. Diagnosis and management of urinary tract infections in adults. BMJ 305:1137-1141, 1992

15b: Vaginitis

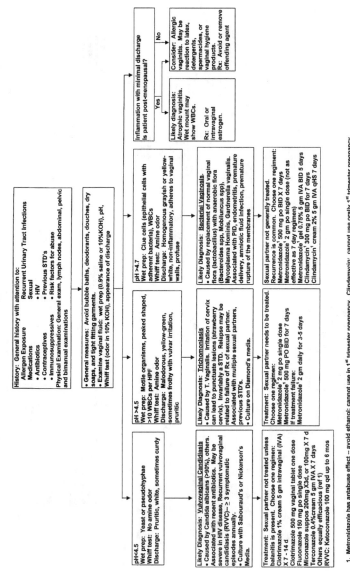

History: General history with attention to:
- Allergen Exposure
- Medications
  - Antibiotics
  - Contraceptives
  - Immunosuppressives
- Recurrent Urinary Tract Infections
- Sexual
  - HIV
  - Previous STD's
  - Risk factors for abuse

Physical Examination: General exam, lymph nodes, abdominal, pelvic and bimanual examinations

- **General measures:** Avoid bubble baths, deodorants, douches, dry soaps, and tight fitting garments.
- **Examine vaginal fluid:** wet prep (0.9% saline or 10%KOH), pH, Whiff test (odor in 10% KOH), appearance of discharge

---

pH<4.5
Wet prep: Yeast or pseudohyphae
Whiff test: No amine odor
Discharge: Pruritic, white, sometimes curdy

Likely Diagnosis: Vulvovaginal Candidiasis
- Caused by Candida albicans (>90%), others. Associated with recent antibiotics. May be severe in HIV disease. Recurrent vulvovaginal candidiasis (RVVC)= ≥ 3 symptomatic episodes annually.
- Culture with Sabouraud's or Nickerson's Media.

Treatment: Sexual partner not treated unless balanitis is present. Choose one regimen:
Clotrimazole 1% cream 5 gm intravaginal (IVA) X 7 - 14 d
Clotrimazole 500 mg vaginal tablet one dose
Fluconazole 150 mg po single dose
Miconazole suppos 200mg X3d, or 100mg X 7 d
Terconazole 0.4%cream 5 gm IVA X 7 days
Others equally efficacious (ref 1)
RVVC: Ketoconazole 100 mg qd up to 6 mos

---

pH >4.5
Wet prep: Motile organisms, peaked shaped, >10 WBCs per HPF
Whiff test: Amine odor
Discharge: Malodorous, yellow-green, sometimes frothy with vulvar irritation, pruritic

Likely Diagnosis: Trichomoniasis
- Caused by T. Vaginalis. Irritation of cervix can lead to punctate lesions (strawberry cervix). Invariably a STD. Relapse may be related to Rx of sexual partner, previous STD's. Associated with multiple sexual partners.
- Culture on Diamond's media.

Treatment: Sexual partner needs to be treated. Choose one regimen:
Metronidazole 2 gm po single dose
Metronidazole 500 mg BID for 7 days
If treatment failure:
Metronidazole 2 gm daily for 3-5 days

---

pH >4.7
Wet prep: Clue cells (epithelial cells with adherent bacterial), WBCs
Whiff test: Amine odor
Discharge: Homogenous grayish or yellow-white, non-inflammatory, adheres to vaginal walls, profuse

Likely Diagnosis: Bacterial Vaginosis.
- Caused by replacement of normal vaginal flora (lactobacillus) with anaerobic flora (Bacteroides spp, Mobiluncus spp), Mycoplasma hominis, Gardnerella vaginalis. Associated with PID, endometritis, premature delivery, amniotic fluid infection, premature rupture of the membranes

Sexual partner not generally treated. Recurrence is common. Choose one regimen:
Metronidazole[1] 500 mg po BID X 7 days
Metronidazole[1] 2 gm po single dose (not as effective as 7 day regimen)
Metronidazole[1] gel 0.75% 5 gm IVA BID 5 days
Clindamycin[1] 300 mg po BID for 7 days
Clindamycin[1] cream 2% 5 gm IVA qHS 7 days

Inflammation with minimal discharge Is patient post-menopausal?

Yes
Likely diagnosis: Atrophic vaginitis. Wet mount may show WBCs.
Rx: Oral or intravaginal estrogen.

No
Consider: Allergic vaginitis. May be reaction to latex, detergents, spermacides, or vaginal hygiene products.
Rx: Avoid or remove offending agent

---

1. Metronidazole has antabuse effect -- avoid ethanol; cannot use in 1st trimester pregnancy. Clindamycin: cannot use orally 1st trimester pregnancy
1998 Guidelines for Treatment of Sexually Transmitted Diseases. MMWR 1998; 47 (No RR-1).
Botash, AS., Howes, D. Vaginitis. June 24, 1998. Http://www.emedicine.aremg/topics631.htm.
Sobol, JD. Candidal Vulvovaginitis. Clinical Obst Gyn 1993; 36: 153-1665.
Fox, KK, Behets, FMT. Vaginal Discharge. Post Grad Med 1995; 98: 87-104.
Easmon, CSF, Hay, PE, Ison, CA. Bacterial Vaginosis: A Diagnostic Approach. Genitourin Med 1992: 68: 134-138.

15c: Urethral Discharge/Genital Ulcers

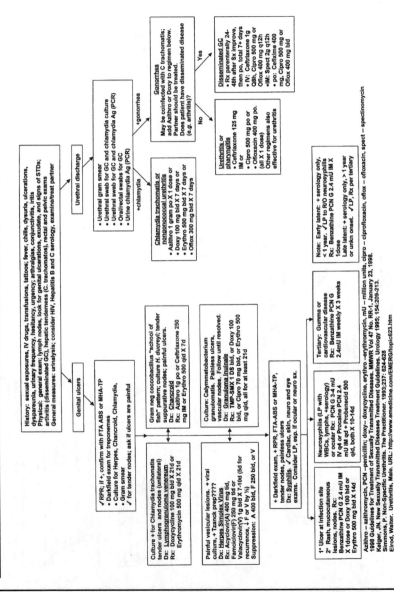

History: sexual exposures, IV drugs, transfusions, tattoos, fever, chills, dysuria, ulcerations, dyspareunia, urinary frequency, hesitancy, urgency; arthralgias, conjunctivitis, iritis
Physical: general exam; lymph nodes, look for genital ulcerations, exudate, and signs of STDs; arthritis (disseminated GC), hepatic tenderness (C. trachomatis), rectal and pelvic exams
General measures: urinalysis; consider HIV, Hepatitis B and C serology, examine/treat partner

Genital ulcers

✓RPR; if +, confirm with FTA ABS or MHA-TP
• Darkfield exam for treponemes
• Culture for Herpes, Chancroid, Chlamydia,
• Gram smear
✓ for tender nodes; ask if ulcers are painful

Culture + for Chlamydia trachomatis tender ulcers and nodes (unilateral)
Dx: **Lymphogranuloma venereum**
Rx: Doxycycline 100 mg bid X 21d or Erythromycin 500 mg qid X 21d

Gram neg coccobacillus "school of fish" pattern; culture *H. ducreyi*; tender suppurative nodes; painful ulcers.
Dx: **Chancroid**
Rx: Azithro 1g po or Ceftriaxone 250 mg IM or Erythro 500 mg qid X 7d

Painful vesicular lesions, + viral culture, + Tzanck prep????
Dx: **Herpes Simplex Virus**
Rx: Acyclovir(A) 400 mg tid,
Famciclovir(F) 250 mg tid or
Valacyclovir(V) 1g bid X 7-10d (3d for recurrence), √ F or V by ⅓)
Suppression: A 400 bid, F 250 bid, or V

Culture: Calymmatobacterium granulomatis. Painless ulcers, vascular nodes. Follow until resolved.
Dx: **Granuloma inguinale**
Rx: TMP/SMX DS bid, or Doxy 100 bid, or Cipro 750 mg bid, or Erythro 500 mg qid, all for at least 21d

+ Darkfield exam, + RPR, FTA-ABS or MHA-TP, tender nodes, painless ulcers
Dx: **Syphilis.** √ Cardiac, skin, neuro and eye exams. Consider LP, esp. if ocular or neuro sx.

1° Ulcer at infection site
2° Rash, mucocutaneous lesions, nodes. Rx:
Benzathine PCN G 2.4 mU IM X 1 dose or Doxy 100 bid or Erythro 500 mg bid X 14d

Neurosyphilis (LP with WBCs, lymphs, +serology) or ocular Rx: PCN G 3-4 mU IV q4 or Procaine PCN 2.4 mU IM qd + Probenecid 500 qid, both X 10-14d

Gumma or cardiovascular disease
Rx: Benzathine PCN G 2.4mU IM weekly X 3 weeks

Tertiary: Gumma or cardiovascular disease
Rx: Benzathine PCN G 2.4mU IM weekly X 3 weeks

Note: Early latent: + serology only, < 1 year. √LP to R/O neurosyphilis
Rx: Benzathine PCN G 2.4 mU IM X 1 dose
Late latent: + serology only, > 1 year or unkn onset. √LP, Rx per tertiary

Urethral discharge

• Urethral gram smear
• Urethral swab for GC and chlamydia culture
• Urethral swab for GC and chlamydia Ag (PCR)
• Oral/rectal swabs for GC
• Urine chlamydia Ag (PCR)

+chlamydia   +gonorrhea

Chlamydia trachomatis or nongonococcal urethritis
• Azithro 1 gram po X 1 dose or
• Doxy 100 mg bid X 7 days or
• Erythro 500 mg bid X 7 days or
• Oflox 300 mg bid X 7 days

Gonorrhea
May be coinfected with C trachomatis; add Azithro or Doxy to regimen below. Partner should be treated. Does patient have disseminated disease (e.g. arthritis)?

No   Yes

Urethritis or pharyngitis
• Ceftriaxone 125 mg IM or
• Cipro 500 mg po or
• Ofloxacin 400 mg po. (all X 1 dose)
Other regimens also effective for urethritis

Disseminated GC
• Rx parenterally 24-48h after Sx improve, then po, total 7+ days
• IV: Ceftriaxone 1g Q8h, Cipro 500 mg q12h or Oflox 400 mg q12h
• IM: Spect 2g q12h
• po: Cefixime 400 mg, Cipro 500 mg or Oflox 400 mg bid

Azithro — azithromycin, PCN — penicillin; doxy — doxycycline, erythro — erythromycin, mU — million units, cipro — ciprofloxacin, oflox — ofloxacin, spect — spectinomycin
1998 Guidelines for Treatment of Sexually Transmitted Diseases. MMWR Vol 47 No. RR-1, January 23, 1998.
Kelger, JN. New Sexually Transmitted Diseases Treatment Guidelines. Urology 1995; 154:209-213.
Simmons, A.R. Non-Specific Urethritis. The Practitioner 1993;237: 624-628
Elrod, Walter. Urethritis, Male. URL: http://www.emedicine.com/EMERG/topic623.htm

15d: Hematuria

Generally defined as greater than 2 RBC's / HPF. Some suggest any RBCs are significant.
- R/O false positive dipstick: hypochlorite, menstrual blood, sexual trauma, medications (chloroquine, L-dopa, methyldopa, nitrofurantoin, phenolphthalein laxatives, phenazopyridine, phenothiazines, pyridium phenytoin, quinine, rifampin), myoglobin, hemoglobin (hemolysis), prophyria, low specific gravity, beets and rhubarb.
- Hx with attention to: trauma, upper respiratory infection (post-streptococcal GN), skin infection (IgA nephropathy), rash/arthritis (SLE), hemoptysis (Goodpasture's, Wegener's), family history (familial hematuria, Alport's [deafness]), sickle cell disease/trait, coagulopathy, urolithiasis, cystic renal disease), porphyria, exercise (benign exercise induced hematuria), medications (anticoagulants,analgesics, cyclophosphamide), renal stones, vasculitis, prior hepatitis B or C, smoker, toxins (bladder tumor), trauma, endometriosis, travel (schistosomiasis), pelvic irradiation.
- PE with attention to ecchymosis, blood pressure (reno-vascular), rash (IgA nephropathy, SLE, Henoch-Schönlein purpura), flank bruit (reno-vascular, A-V fistula), evidence of endocarditis, BPH

No dx made by H & P

Is gross hematuria present?

No → Urine dipstick and microscopic analysis

- **RBCs with crystals** → See Kidney Stones
- **Dysmorphic RBCs with RBC casts and proteinuria** → Likely glomerular source. √ ANA, ANCA, ASO, anti-GBM Ab, cryoglobulins, C3, C4, anti-ds DNA, HIV, VDRL. See Evaluation of suspected vasculitis. • Consult Nephrology to consider renal biopsy.
- **RBCs with WBCs and bacteria** → Likely dx: Urinary tract infection. See Urinary Tract Infections → Recheck urinalysis → pyuria → √ urine AFB and PPD to R/O TB. / hematuria → (see RBCs without casts) / normal → No further workup
- **RBCs without casts, crystals, or bacteria** → Renal and bladder ultrasound → positive → Treat / negative → Is age > 40? → no → √ 24h urine to R/O hyperuricosuria and hypercalciuria. • If negative, √IVP, urine cytology. / yes → • √IVP, urine cytology to R/O tumors • If negative, cystoscopy (esp. smokers) • If negative, CT with contrast • If negative, 24h urine to R/O hyperuricosuria and hypercalciuria.
  - → negative workup → • Consider renal biopsy • Recheck urinalysis and cytology q 6 mos and cystoscopy/ IVP q 12 mos X 3 years.

Yes → 3 glass test (fill 3 glasses sequentially from a single void) or relation of hematuria to urine flow
- **All 3 glasses or Throughout urine stream** → Lesion in bladder, ureter(s), or kidney(s) → (see RBCs without casts / Renal and bladder ultrasound)
- **1st glass or Beginning of stream** → Likely urethral source. Consult Urology for cystoscopy
- **3rd glass or Termination of stream** → Likely posterior urethra, bladder neck or prostate source → Consult Urology for cystoscopy and/or prostate evaluation

Schaeffer AJ, Del Greco F. Other renal diseases of urologic significance. In: Walsh, PC, Retik, AB, Stamey, TA, Vaughan, ED (ed), Campbell's Urology, pp 2065-72, W. B. Saunders 1992.
Kanarvogel, LE. Common urinary symptoms: Hematuria. In: Rakel, RE (editor), Sanders Manual of Medical Practice, pp 518-519. W. B. Saunders, 1996
Ahmed Z, Lee J. Asymptomatic urinary abnormalities: Hematuria and Proteinuria. Med Clin NA 1997: 81: 641-649
Sparwasser C, Cimniak HU, Treiber U, Pust RA. Significance of the evaluation of asymptomatic microscopic haematuria in young men. BJ Urol 1994; 74: 723-729.
Rockall AG, Newman-Sanders APG, Al-Kutoubi MA, Vale JA. Haematuria. Postgrad Med J 1997; 73: 129-136
Fracchia JA, Motta J, Miller LS, et al. Evaluation of asymptomatic microhematuria. Urology 1995; 46:484-489.

15e: Lower Urinary Tract Symptoms and Benign Prostatic Hyperplasia (BPH)

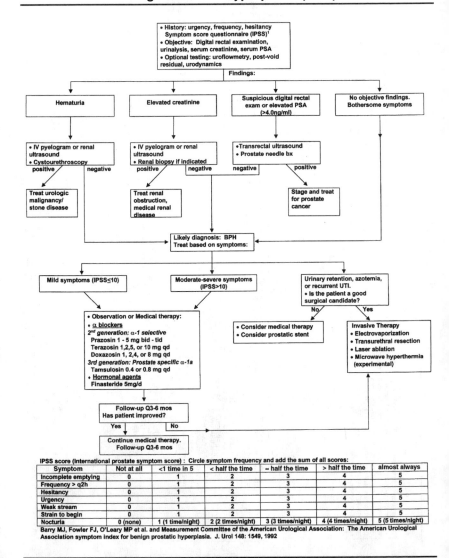

- History: urgency, frequency, hesitancy
  Symptom score questionnaire (IPSS)[1]
- Objective: Digital rectal examination, urinalysis, serum creatinine, serum PSA
- Optional testing: uroflowmetry, post-void residual, urodynamics

Findings:

Hematuria
- IV pyelogram or renal ultrasound
- Cystourethroscopy
  - positive → Treat urologic malignancy/stone disease
  - negative

Elevated creatinine
- IV pyelogram or renal ultrasound
- Renal biopsy if indicated
  - positive → Treat renal obstruction, medical renal disease
  - negative

Suspicious digital rectal exam or elevated PSA (>4.0ng/ml)
- Transrectal ultrasound
- Prostate needle bx
  - negative
  - positive → Stage and treat for prostate cancer

No objective findings. Bothersome symptoms

Likely diagnosis: BPH
Treat based on symptoms:

Mild symptoms (IPSS≤10)

Moderate-severe symptoms (IPSS>10)

Urinary retention, azotemia, or recurrent UTI.
- Is the patient a good surgical candidate?
  - No →
    - Consider medical therapy
    - Consider prostatic stent
  - Yes → Invasive Therapy
    - Electrovaporization
    - Transurethral resection
    - Laser ablation
    - Microwave hyperthermia (experimental)

- Observation or Medical therapy:
- α blockers
  2nd generation: α-1 selective
  Prazosin 1 - 5 mg bid - tid
  Terazosin 1,2,5, or 10 mg qd
  Doxazosin 1, 2,4, or 8 mg qd
  3rd generation: Prostate specific α-1a
  Tamsulosin 0.4 or 0.8 mg qd
- Hormonal agents
  Finasteride 5mg/d

Follow-up Q3-6 mos
Has patient improved?
- Yes → Continue medical therapy. Follow-up Q3-6 mos
- No

IPSS score (International prostate symptom score) : Circle symptom frequency and add the sum of all scores:

Symptom	Not at all	<1 time in 5	< half the time	≈ half the time	> half the time	almost always
Incomplete emptying	0	1	2	3	4	5
Frequency > q2h	0	1	2	3	4	5
Hesitancy	0	1	2	3	4	5
Urgency	0	1	2	3	4	5
Weak stream	0	1	2	3	4	5
Strain to begin	0	1	2	3	4	5
Nocturia	0 (none)	1 (1 time/night)	2 (2 times/night)	3 (3 times/night)	4 (4 times/night)	5 (5 times/night)

Barry MJ, Fowler FJ, O'Leary MP et al. and Measurement Committee of the American Urological Association: The American Urological Association symptom index for benign prostatic hyperplasia. J. Urol 148: 1549, 1992

16a: Dosing and Renal Failure Adjustments for Commonly Prescribed Drugs

Dosing and renal adjustments for some commonly used agents are listed below. Doses within an antibiotic range should be chosen based on severity. For antihypertensives and oral diabetic agents, start at the low end of the range. Check references for additional information and other agents. Supplementation for hemodialysis patients are listed in column 6 when applicable. Dose ranges are guidelines only; dosages may need to be adjusted by drug level and clinical effect where appropriate.
- GFR can be estimated using the Cockcroft/Gault formula: [(140-age) X ideal body weight in kg]/(72 X serum creatinine in mg/dl). Multiply by 0.85 for females. Formula can only be used if creatinine is stable. Assume oliguric patients to have a creatinine clearance < 10.
- Ideal body weight for men = 50 kg for first 5 feet, plus 2.3 kg for each additional inch.
- Ideal body weight for women = 45.5 kg for first 5 feet, plus 2.3 kg for each additional inch.

Antibiotics

1. Aminoglycosides

Drug	Normal	GFR > 50	GFR 10-50	GFR<10	Hemodialysis supplement
Amikacin/ Kanamycin	5 mg/kg q8h	3 - 4.5 mg/kg q12h	1.5 - 3.5 mg/kg q12 - 18 h	1 - 1.5 mg/kg q24 - 48 h	3.5 mg/kg post dialysis
Gentamicin/ Tobramycin	1 - 1.5 mg/kg q8h	0.5 - 1 mg/kg q8-12h	0.3 - 0.7 mg/kg q12h	0.2-0.3 mg/kg q24-48h	0.7 mg/kg post dialysis
Streptomycin	1g qd	1 g qd	1g q24-72h	1g q72-96h	0.5 g post dialysis

2. Cephalosporins

Drug	Normal	GFR > 50	GFR 10-50	GFR<10	Hemodialysis supplement
Cefaclor	250 - 500 mg q8h or 375 - 500 mg extended release q12h	250 - 500 mg q8h or 375 - 500 mg extended release q12h	250 500 mg q8h or 375 - 500 mg extended release q12h	250 mg q8h or 375 mg extended release q12h	250 mg post dialysis
Cefadroxil	500 - 1000 mg q12h	500 - 1000 mg q12h	500 - 1000 mg q12 - 24h	500 - 1000 mg q12h	500 - 1000 mg post dialysis
Cefamandole	500 - 1000 mg q4 - 6h	500 - 1000 mg q6h	500 - 1000 mg q6 - 8h	500 - 1000 mg q12h	500 - 1000 mg post dialysis
Cefazolin	500 - 1500 mg q6h	500 - 1500 mg q8h	500 - 1500 mg q12h	500 - 1500 mg q24 - 48h	500 - 1000 mg post dialysis
Cefepime	250 - 2000 mg q8h	250 - 2000 mg q12h	250 - 2000 mg q12 - 16h	250 - 2000 mg q24 - 48h	1000 mg post dialysis
Cefixime	200 mg q12h or 400 mg qd	200 mg q12h or 400 mg qd	300 mg qd	200 mg qd	300 mg post dialysis
Cefonicid	1g qd	500 mg qd	500 - 500 mg qd	100 mg qd	none
Cefotaxime	1 - 2 g q4 - 6h	1 - 2 g q6h	1 - 2 g q8 - 12h (PDR suggests half of normal dose if GFR<20)	1 - 2 g q24h (PDR suggests half of normal dose if GFR<20)	1 gram after dialysis
Cefotetan	1 - 2 g q12h	1 - 2 g q12h	1 - 2 g q24h (GFR < 30)	1 - 2 g q48h	1 gram after dialysis
Cefoxitin	1 - 2 g q6-8h	1 - 2 g q8h	1 - 2 g q8-12h	1 - 2 g q24-48h	1 gram after dialysis
Cefpodoxime	200 mg q12h	200 mg q12h	200 mg q16h	200 mg q24 - 48h	200 mg after dialysis
Ceftazidime	1 - 2 g q8h	1 - 2 g q8 - 12h	1 - 2 g q24 - 48h	1 - 2 g q48h	1 gram after dialysis
Ceftizoxime	1 - 2 g q8 - 12h	1 - 2 g q8 - 12h	1 - 2 g q12 - 24h	1 - 2 g qd	1 gram after dialysis
Cefuroxime sodium	750 - 1500 mg q8h	750 - 1500 mg q8h	750 mg q12h (GFR -20)	750 mg qd	Dose after dialysis
Cephalexin/ Cephradine	250 - 500 mg q8h	250 - 500 mg q8h	250 - 500 mg q12h	250 - 500 mg q24h	Dose after dialysis

No renal adjustment necessary: Cefaperazone (1- 2g q12h), Ceftriaxone (1 - 2 g qd; or 2 g q12h for meningitis), Cefuroxime axetil (250 - 500 mg q12h)

3. Macrolides/azalides

Drug	Normal	GFR > 50	GFR 10-50	GFR<10	Hemodialysis supplement
Clarithromycin	500 - 1000 mg q12h	500 - 1000 mg q12h	500 - 750 mg q12h	250 - 750 mg q12h	Dose after hemolysis
Erythromycin	250 - 500 mg q6-12h	250 - 1000 mg q6-12h	250 - 1000 mg q6-12h	250 - 750 mg q6-12h	None

No renal adjustment necessary: Azithromycin (500 mg day 1, then 250 - 500 mg qd)

16a: Dosing and Renal Failure Adjustments for Commonly Prescribed Drugs (continued)

4. Penicillins

Drug	Normal	GFR > 50	GFR 10-50	GFR<10	Hemodialysis dose
Amoxicillin	250-500 mg q8h	250 - 500 mg q8h	250 - 500 mg q8-12h	250 - 500 mg qd	250 - 500 mg post dialysis
Ampicillin	250 mg - 2 g q6h	250 mg - 2 g q6h	250 mg - 2 g q6 - 12h	250 mg - 2 g q12-24h	250 mg - 2 g post dialysis
Amoxicillin/clavulanic acid	250 mg q8h or 500 - 875 mg q12h	250 mg q8h or 500 - 875 mg q12h	250 - 500 mg q12h	250 - 500 mg qd	250 - 500 mg during and post dialysis
Ampicillin/sulbactam	1.5 - 3 g q6h	1.5 - 3 g q6h	1.5 - 3 g q8 - 12h	1.5 - 3 g qd	1.5 3 g post dialysis
Methicillin	1 - 2 g q4h	1 - 2 g q4 - 6h	1 - 2 g q6 - 8h	1 - 2 g q8 - 12h	none
Mezlocillin	1.5 - 4.0 g q 4 - 6h	1.5 - 4.0 g q 4 - 6h	1.5 - 4.0 g q 4 - 6h	1.5 - 4.0 g q 8 - 12h	none
Penicillin G	0.5 - 4 million U q6h	0.5 - 4 million U q6h	0.375 - 3 million U q6h	0.2 - 2 million U q6h	0.5 - 4 million U post dialysis
Piperacillin	3 - 4 g q6h	3 - 4 g q4 - 6h	3 - 4 g q6 - 8h	3 - 4 g q8h	3 - 4 g post dialysis
Piperacillin/tazobactam	3.375 g q4-6h	3.375 g q6h	2.25 g q6h (GFR 20-50)	2.25 g 8 (GFR < 20)	2.25 q8, + 0.75 g post dialysis
Ticarcillin	3 g q4h	1 - 2g q4h	1 - 2g q4h	1 - 2g q12h	3g post dialysis
Ticarcillin/ clavulanic acid	3.1 g q4 - 6h	3.1 g q4 - 6h	2g q4 h (GFR 30 -60) 2 g q8h (GFR 10 - 30)	2g q12h	3.1 g post dialysis

No renal adjustment necessary: Nafcillin (1-2g q4-6h), Penicillin VK (250 - 500 mg q6h)

5. Quinolones

Drug	Normal	GFR > 50	GFR 10-50	GFR<10	Hemodialysis supplement
Ciprofloxacin	500- 750 mg q 12h po OR 200 – 400 mg q 12h IV	500- 750 mg q 12h po OR 200 – 400 mg q 12h IV	250- 500 mg q 12h po OR 200 – 400 mg q 18 - 24h IV (GFR < 30)	250 - 375 mg q 12h po OR 200 – 400 mg q 18 - 24h IV	250 mg q12h po
Levofloxacin	250 - 500 mg qd (IV or po)	250 - 500 mg qd (IV or po)	500 mg load, then 250 mg qd (IV or po, GFR 20 - 50)	500 mg load, then 250 mg q48h (IV or po, GFR < 20)	Dose per GFR < 10, no supplement needed
Norfloxacin	400 mg po q12h	400 mg po q12h	400 mg po q12 - 24h	Avoid	Avoid
Ofloxacin	400 mg q 24	200 mg qd	100 - 200 mg qd		

No renal adjustment necessary: Trovofloxacin (100 – 200 mg po qd), Alatrofloxacin (200 – 300 mg IV qd)

6. Tetracyclines

Drug	Normal	GFR > 50	GFR 10-50	GFR<10	Hemodialysis supplement
Tetracycline	250 - 500 mg qd	250 - 500 mg q8-12h	250 - 500 mg q12 - 24h	250 - 500 mg qd	no supplement

No renal adjustment necessary: Minocycline (100 mg q12h), Doxycycline (100 mg qd)

7. Miscellaneous antibacterials

Drug	Normal	GFR > 50	GFR 10-50	GFR<10	Hemodialysis supplement
Aztreonam	1 - 2 g q6-12h	1 - 2 g q6-12h	1 - 2 g load, then 0.5 - 1g q 8 - 12h (GFR 10 - 30)	1 - 2 g load, then 250 - 500 mg q6-12h	0.5g post dialysis
Imipenem	250 - 1000 mg q6h	250 - 1000 mg q6h	250 - 500 mg q8h	250 mg q6h	Dose post dialysis
Metronidazole	7.5 mg/kg q6h	7.5 mg/kg q6h	7.5 mg/kg q6h	3.75 mg/kg q6h	Dose post dialysis
Nitrofurantoin	50 – 100 mg q6h	50 – 100 mg q6h	Avoid	Avoid	Avoid
Trimethoprim/sulfisoxazole (severe UTI or Shigella)	8 - 10 mg/kg/day (based on TMP) divided in equal q 6 to q12h doses	8 - 10 mg/kg/day (based on TMP) divided in equal q 6 to q12h doses	4 - 5 mg/kg/day (based on TMP) divided in equal q8 to q12h doses (GFR < 30)	Avoid	Avoid
Trimethoprim/sulfisoxazole (Pneumocystis carinii)	15 - 20 mg/kg/day (based on TMP) divided in equal q8 or q6h doses	15 - 20 mg/kg/day (based on TMP) divided in equal q8 or q6h doses	7.5 - 10 mg/kg/d (based on TMP) divided in equal q8 or q6h doses (GFR < 30)	Avoid	Avoid
Vancomycin	500 mg q6h or 1g q12h	500 mg q6-12h	500mg q24-48h	500 mg q48-96h or 1 g q7d, adjust dose for drug levels	

No renal adjustment necessary: Chloramphenicol (12.5 mg/kg q6h), Clindamycin (150 - 300 mg q6h)

8. Antifungals

Drug	Normal	GFR > 50	GFR 10-50	GFR<10	Hemodialysis supplement
Amphotericin B	20 – 40 mg (or 0.25-1.5 mg/kg) qd	20 – 40 mg (or 0.25-1.5 mg/kg/d	20 – 40 mg (or 0.25-1.5 mg/kg) qd	20 – 40 mg (or 0.25-1.5 mg/kg) q24-36h	none
Amphotericin B lipid complex	Abelcet 5 mg/kg qd; Amphotec 3 - 4 mg/kg qd	Recommendations not available	Recommendations not available	Recommendations not available	
Flucytosine	37.5 mg/kg q6h	37.5 mg/kg q12h	37.5 mg/kg q16h	37.5 mg/kg qd	Dose after dialysis
Itraconazole	100 - 200 mg q12h	100 - 200 mg q12h	100 - 200 mg q12h	50 - 100 mg q12h	none

No renal adjustment necessary: Fluconazole (200 -400 mg qd; 200 mg after dialysis), Ketoconazole (200 mg qd), Miconazole (200 - 1200 mg q8h)

Antiviral agents

Drug	Normal	GFR > 50	GFR 10-50	GFR <10	Hemodialysis supplement
Acyclovir	5 mg/kg q8h	5 mg/kg q8h	5 mg/kg q12-24h	2.5 mg/kg q24h	2.5 mg/kg post HD
Didanosine	≥ 60 mg: 200 mg q12h; < 60 mg: 125 mg q12h	Recommendations not available	Recommendations not available	Recommendations not available	Recommendations not available
Ganciclovir (Induction IV)	5 mg/kg q12h	2.5 mg/kg q12h	2.5 mg/kg q24h (GFR 25-49); 1.25 mg/kg q24h (GFR 10-24)	1.25 mg/kg TIW	1.25 mg/kg TIW post dialysis
(Maintenance IV)	5 mg/kg q24h	2.5 mg/kg q24h	1.25 mg/kg q24h (GFR 25-49); 0.625 mg/kg q24h (GFR 10-24)	0.625 mg/kg TIW	0.625 mg/kg TIW post dialysis
(PO)	1000 mg q8h	500 mg q8h	500mg q12h (GFR 25-49); 500 mg q24h (GFR 10-24)	500 mg TIW	500 mg TIW post dialysis
Lamivudine	150 mg q12h	150 mg q12h	150 mg x1, then 100 mg qd (GFR 30-49); 150 mg x1, then 50 mg qd (GFR 15-29)	150 mg x1, then 50 mg qd (GFR 5-14); 50 mg x1 then 25 mg qd (GFR <5)	No recommendations
Nevirapine	200 mg q12h	Recommendations not available	Recommendations not available	Recommendations not available	Recommendations not available
Stavudine	≥ 60 kg: 40 mg q12h; < 60 kg: 30 mg q12h	≥ 60 kg: 40 mg q12h; < 60 kg: 30 mg q12h	≥ 60 kg: 20 mg q12h (GFR 26-50); < 60 kg: 15 mg q12h (GFR 26-50); ≥ 60 kg: 20 mg q24h (GFR 10-25); < 60 kg: 15 mg q24h (GFR 10-25)	Recommendations not available	Recommendations not available
Zalcitibine	0.75 mg q8h	0.75 mg q8h (GFR >40)	0.75 mg q12h (GFR 10-40)	0.75 mg q24h	Recommendations not available
Zidovudine	200 mg q8h	200 mg q8h	Recommendations not available	Recommendations not available	100 mg q8h

No renal adjustment necessary: Indinavir (800 mg q8h), Nelfinavir (750 mg q8h), Ritonavir (600 mg q12h), Saquinavir (Invirase 600 mg q8h pc; Fortovase 1200mg q8h pc)

16a: Dosing and Renal Failure Adjustments for Commonly Prescribed Drugs (continued)

Antihypertensive and Cardiovascular drugs

1. Adrenergic/serotinergic mediators

Drug	Normal	GFR > 50	GFR 10-50	GFR<10	Hemodialysis supplement
Guanadrel	10 - 50 mg q12h	10 - 50 mg q12h	10 - 50 mg q12 -24h	10 - 50 mg q24 - 48h	unknown
Guanethidine	10 - 100 mg qd	10 - 100 mg qd	10 - 100 mg qd	10 - 100 mg q 24 - 46h	unknown
Methyldopa	250 - 500 mg q 8h	250 - 500 mg q 8h	250 - 500 mg q 8 - 12h	250 - 500 mg q 12 - 24h	250 mg post dialysis
Reserpine	0.05 - 0.25 mg qd	0.05 - 0.25 mg qd	0.05 - 0.25 mg qd	avoid	avoid

No renal adjustment necessary: Clonidine (0.1 to 0.6 mg q12h, or TTS 1, 2, or 3 patch q week), Doxazosin (1 - 16 mg qd), Guanabenz (8 - 16 mg q12h), Ketanserin (40 mg q12h),
Prazosin (1 - 15 mg q12h), Terazosin (1 - 20 mg qd)

2. Angiotensin converting enzyme inhibitors/Angiotensin II receptor antagonists

Drug	Normal	GFR > 50	GFR 10-50	GFR<10	Hemodialysis supplement
Benazepril	10 - 40 mg qd	10 - 40 mg qd	5 - 40 mg qd	5 - 20 mg qd	5 mg
Captopril	25 - 50 mg q8 - 12h	25 - 50 mg q8 - 12h	12.5 - 25 mg q12 - 18h	12.5 mg qd	6.25 mg post dialysis
Enalapril	5 - 40 mg qd	5 - 40 mg qd	2.5 - 40 mg qd	2.5 - 40 mg qd	2.5 - 10 mg
Fosinopril	10 - 40 mg qd	10 - 40 mg qd	10 - 40 mg qd	10 - 30 mg qd	none
Lisinopril	10 - 40 mg qd	10 - 40 mg qd	5 - 40 mg qd	2.5 - 40 mg qd	2.5 - 10 mg post dialysis
Quinapril	10 - 20 mg qd	10 - 20 mg qd	2.5 - 5 mg qd	2.5 - 5 mg qd	2.5 mg post dialysis
Ramipril	2.5 - 20 mg qd	2.5 - 20 mg qd	1.25 - 5 mg qd	1.25 - 5 mg qd	1.25

No renal adjustment necessary: Losartan (25 - 100 mg qd), valsartan (80 - 320 mg qd)

3. Beta adrenergic blockers

Drug	Normal	GFR > 50	GFR 10-50	GFR<10	Hemodialysis supplement
Acebutolol	200 -800 mg qd (or divide bid)	200 -800 mg qd (or divide bid)	200 -400 mg qd (or divide bid)	200 mg qd	none
Atenolol	50 - 100 mg qd	50 - 100 mg qd	50 mg q24 - 48h	25 mg q24 - 96h	25 - 50 mg
Betaxolol	10 - 20 mg qd	10 - 20 mg qd	10 - 20 mg qd	5 - 10 mg qd	none
Carteolol	2.5 - 10 mg qd	2.5 - 10 mg qd	2.5 - 10 mg q 48h	2.5 - 10 mg q 72h	

No renal adjustment necessary: Esmolol (50 - 150 µg/kg/min infusion), Labetalol (200 - 600 mg q 12h), Metoprolol (50 - 100 mg q12h), Penbutolol (10 - 40 mg qd), Pindolol (10 - 40 mg qd), Propranalol (20 - 160 mg q 12h), Timolol (10 - 20 mg q12h)

4. Central agents

Drug	Normal	GFR > 50	GFR 10-50	GFR<10	Hemodialysis supplement
Clonidine/chlorthalidone	Clonidine 0.1 - 0.3 mg/ Chlorthalidone 15 mg bid	Clonidine 0.1 - 0.3 mg/ Chlorthalidone 15 mg bid	Clonidine 0.1 - 0.3 mg/ Chlorthalidone 15 mg qd (adjustment for diuretic)	Clonidine 0.1 - 0.3 mg/ Chlorthalidone 15 mg q48 (adjustment for diuretic)	Contraindicated for anuria. Use alternative agent.
Methyldopa	250 -500 mg q6 -12 h (250 bid if used in combination with a non- thiazide antihypertensive)	250 - 500 mg qd	250 - 500 mg q 8 - 12h	250 - 500 mg q 12 - 24 h	250 mg post dialysis

No renal adjustment necessary:

Drug	Normal	GFR > 50	GFR 10-50	Normal
Clonidine	0.1 - 0.3 mg bid (1.2 mg bid is rarely used, maximum dose)	Clonidine 0.1 - 0.3 mg/ Chlorthalidone 15 mg bid	Guanfacine	1 - 2 mg qhs
Clonidine TTS	TTS - 1, TTS - 2, TTS - 3. Programmed delivery of 0.1, 0.2, or 0.3 mg clonidine per day for one week. Apply 1 - 2 patches weekly; adjust dose to BP.			

16a: Dosing and Renal Failure Adjustments for Commonly Prescribed Drugs (continued)

5. Vasodilators

Drug	Normal	GFR > 50	GFR 10-50	GFR<10	Hemodialysis supplement
Hydralazine	25 - 50 mg q8h	25 - 50 mg q8h	25 - 50 mg q8h	25 - 50 mg q8 - 16h	none

No renal adjustment necessary: Diazoxide 150 - 300 mg q bolus, Minoxidil 5 - 30 mg q 12h, Nitroprusside 0.25 - 8 μg/kg/min infusion

6. Calcium Channel Blockers

No renal adjustments necessary:

Drug (dihydropyridine)	Normal
Amlodipine	5 - 10 mg qd
Felodipine sustained release	2.5 - 10 mg qd
Isradipine	5 - 10 mg qd
Nicardipine	20 - 30 mg q 8h
Nifedipine	10 - 30 mg q 8h or
	30 - 120 mg qd (sustained release)
Nimodipine	30 mg q 8h
Nisoldipine sustained release ?	20 - 60 mg qd

Drug (non-dihydropyridine)	Normal
Diltiazem	30 mg q6h to 120 mg q6 - 8h
Diltiazem sustained release	90 – 180 mg q12 or 180 – 480 mg qd (depending on preparation)
Verapamil	80 - 120 mg q 8h
Verapamil sustained release	180 mg q 24 - 240 mg q 12h

6. Oral antiarrhythmic agents

Drug	Normal	GFR > 50	GFR 10-50	GFR<10	Hemodialysis supplement
Disopyramide	100 - 200 mg q6h or 200 - 300 mg extended release q12	100 - 200 mg q8h	100 - 200 mg q12 - 24h	100 - 200 mg q24 -40h	None
Flecainide	50 - 200 mg q 12h	50 - 200 mg q 12h	50 mg q 12h, adjust by level	50 mg q 12h or 100 mg qd, adjust by level	None
Mexiletine	150 - 300 mg q6-12h	150 - 300 mg q6-12h	150 - 300 mg q6-12h	150 - 250 mg q6-12h	None
Procainamide	25 mg/kg extended release q12h	25 mg/kg extended release q12h	350 - 400 mg regular procainamide q6 - 12h	350 - 400 mg regular procainamide q8 - 24h	200 mg
Quinidine	200 - 400 mg q 4 - 6h	200 - 400 mg q 4 - 6h	200 - 400 mg q 4 - 6h	200 - 300 mg q 4 - 6h	200 mg
Sotalol	80 - 160 mg q12h	80 - 160 mg q12h	80 - 160 mg q24 - 48h	individualize	80 mg
Tocainide	400 - 600 mg q6h	400 - 600 mg q6h	400 - 600 mg q8h	200 - 400 mg q 8h	200 mg

No renal adjustment necessary: Moricizine (200 - 300 mg q8h), Propafenone (150 - 300 mg q8h)
Oral anti-arrhythmic agents should be adjusted to drug level and effect and should be prescribed by physicians familiar with their use.

Non-sedating antihistamines

Drug	Normal	GFR > 50	GFR 10-50	GFR<10	Hemodialysis supplement
Cetirizine	5 - 20 mg qd	5 - 10 mg qd	5 mg qd (GFR < 30)	5 mg qd	none
Fexofenadine	60 mg q 12h	60 mg q 12h	60 mg q 12 - 24h	60 mg qd	none
Loratadine	10 mg qd	10 mg qd	10 mg q 48h (GFR < 30)	10 mg q 48h	none

No renal adjustment necessary: Astemizole (10 mg qd)

Gastrointestinal agents

1. H-2 blockers

Drug	Normal	GFR > 50	GFR 10-50	GFR<10	Hemodialysis supplement
Cimetidine	400 mg q 12h or 400 - 800 mg qhs	400 mg q12h or 400 - 800 mg qhs	300 mg q12h	200 mg hs to 300 mg q12	none

135

Famotidine	20 - 40 mg qhs	20 mg qhs	20 mg qhs	20 mg q 24 - 48h	none
Nizatidine	150 - 300 mg qhs	150 - 300 mg qhs	150 mg qhs (GFR >20) maintenance: q 48h	150 mg q 48h (GFR<20) maintenance: q 72h	none
Ranitidine	150 q 12h or 300 mg qhs	150 q 12h or 300 mg qhs	150 mg qhs	150 mg qhs	time doses for post-dialysis

2. Proton pump inhibitors

No renal adjustment necessary: Lansoprazole (15 - 30 mg qd), Omeprazole (20 - 40 mg qd)

Oral Hypoglycemic agents

Drug	Normal	GFR > 50	GFR 10-50	GFR<10	Hemodialysis supplement
Acarbose	25 - 100 mg tid at start of meal	Avoid if creatinine > 2	Avoid	Avoid	
Acetohexamide	250 - 1500 mg qd	Avoid	Avoid	Avoid	
Chlorpropamide	100 - 500 mg qd	100 - 250 mg qd	Avoid	Avoid	
Glimepiride	1-8 mg qd	1-8 mg qd	1 mg qd (GFR<22)	1 mg qd	
Glyburide	1.25 - 20 mg qd (or divide bid)	Unknown	Avoid	Avoid	
Metformin	500 - 1000 mg bid with meals	Avoid	Avoid	Avoid	

No renal adjustment necessary: Glipizide (5 - 20 mg qd before breakfast), Tolazamide (100 - 250 mg qd before breakfast), Tolbutamide (1 - 2 g qd before breakfast), Troglitazone 200 – 600 mg qd.
Adjust doses based on serum glucose and q 3 month HbA1C levels. See *Management of Diabetes*

Anticonvulsant agents
See *Management of Status Epilepticus* for intravenous dosing

Drug	Normal	GFR > 50	GFR 10-50	GFR<10	Hemodialysis supplement
Gabapentin	300 - 800 mg qd. Start 300 mg day 1, bid day 2, tid day 3.	400 mg q8h (GFR < 60)	300 mg q12h (GFR 30 - 60) 300 mg qd (GFR 14 - 30)	300 mg q48h	200 - 300 mg post each 4 hours of dialysis
Primidone	250 - 500 mg q6 - 8h. Start at 100 mg qhs day 1-3, then increase over 9 days.	250 - 500 mg q8h	250 - 500 mg q8-12h	250 - 500 mg q12-24h	1/3 dose
Topiramate	200 - 800 mg q12h. Start at 50 mg qhs, increase over 8 weeks	50% of usual dose (GFR < 70)	50% of usual dose		Supplemental dose post dialysis

Drug	Normal
Phenytoin	1000 mg load, then 200 - 400 mg qd
Valproic acid	15 - 60 mg/kg/d. If >250 mg, divide bid.

No renal adjustments necessary:

Drug	Normal
Carbamazepine	200 mg q12h to 400 tid or 600 mg q12(XR)
Ethosuximide	500 - 1500 mg qd
Felbamate	400 - 1200 mg tid

Bennett WM et al. Drug Prescribing in Renal Failure: Dosing guidelines for adults, 3rd ed. American College of Physicians, Philadelphia. 1994
Physicians Desk Reference. Medical Economics Co, Montvale NJ. 1998
Micromedex

16b: Infusions Commonly Used in the ICU

DRUG	USUAL DOSE	STANDARD DILUTION [concentrated dilution]	STANDARD CONCENTRATION [concentrated]	SOLUTION	RATE (ml/hr) (ml/kg/hr)# [concentrated]	MAXIMUM DOSE
Amiodarone HCl	Bolus: 150mg over 10 min Infuse: (1) 1 mg/min for 6 hr; then (2) 0.5 mg/min	Bolus: 150 mg/100ml 900mg/500ml	Bolus: 1.5 mg/ml Drip: 1.8 mg/ml	D5W only	Bolus: 600 (1) 33.3; (2)16.7	1 mg/min
Aminone Lactate	Bolus: 0.75mg/kg over 2-3 min Infuse: 5-20 mcg/kg/min	500mg/250ml	2 mg/ml	NSS only	Varies	18 mg/kg/day
Bretylium	Bolus: 5 mg/kg then 10 mg/kg up to total of 30; Infuse: 1-2 mg/min	1000mg/250ml	4 mg/ml	D5W or NSS	15-30	40 mg/kg/day
Bumetanide	1-4 mg/hr	24mg/96ml	0.25 mg/ml	Undiluted	4-16	8 mg/hr
Cisatracurium Besylate	Bolus: 0.15-0.2 mg/kg Infuse: 1-5 mcg/kg/min (0.06-0.3 mg/kg/hr)	400mg/200ml	2 mg/ml	D5W or NSS	0.03-0.15#	Titrate
Cyclosporin	1/3 usual oral dose over 24 hr	100ml	Varies	D5W	Varies	Varies
Diazepam	5-10 mg/hr	50mg/250ml [500mg/100ml]	0.2 mg/ml [5 mg/ml]	NSS [Undiluted]	25-50 [1-2]	Titrate
Diltiazem HCl	5-15 mg/hr	125mg/125ml	1 mg/ml	D5W or NSS	5-15	15 mg/hr
Dobutamine HCl	2.5-20 mcg/kg/min (0.15-1.2 mg/kg/hr)	500mg/250ml [1000mg/250ml]	2 mg/ml [4 mg/ml]	D5W or NSS	0.075-0.6# [0.0375-0.3]	40 mcg/kg/min
Dopamine HCl	1-20 mcg/kg/min (0.06-1.2 mg/kg/hr)	400mg/250ml [3200mg/250ml]	1.6 mg/ml [12.8 mg/ml]	D5W or NSS	0.0375-0.75# [0.0047-0.094]	40 mcg/kg/min
Epinephrine HCl	1-10 mcg/min	2 mg/250ml [16mg/250ml]	0.008mg/ml [0.064 mg/ml]	D5W or NSS	7.5-75 [0.94-9.4]	20 mcg/min
Esmolol HCl	Bolus: 500 mcg/kg Infuse: 50-200 mcg/kg/min (3-12 mg/kg/hr)	5000mg/500ml [10,000mg/500ml]	10 mg/ml [20 mg/ml]	D5W or NSS	0.3-1.2# [0.15-0.6]	300 mcg/kg/min
Fentanyl Citrate	0.02-0.08 mcg/kg/min (0.0012-0.0048 mg/kg/hr)	2mg/250ml [4mg/250ml]	0.008 mg/ml [0.016 mg/ml]	D5W or NSS	0.15-0.6# [0.075-0.3]	Titrate
Furosemide	10-80 mg/hr	1000mg/100ml	10 mg/ml	Undiluted	1-8	240 mg/hr
Glucagon	1-5 mg/hr	Varies	Varies	D5W or NSS	Varies	5 mg/hr

16b: Infusions Commonly Used in the ICU (continued)

DRUG	USUAL DOSE	STANDARD DILUTION [concentrated dilution]	STANDARD CONCENTRATION [concentrated]	SOLUTION	RATE (ml/hr)# [(ml/kg/hr)# [concentrated]	MAXIMUM DOSE
Haloperidol Lactate	10 mg/hr	200mg/200ml [200mg/100ml]	1 mg/ml [2 mg/ml]	D5W	10 [5]	Titrate
Heparin Sodium	500-3200 Units/hr	25,000 Units/250ml	100 Units/ml	D5W or NSS	5-32	Titrate
Hydromorphone HCl	0.2-2 mg/hr	1 mg/ml [4 mg/ml]	1 mg/ml [4 mg/ml]	Undiluted	0.2-2 [0.05-0.5]	Titrate
Insulin Regular	0.1-0.2 Units/kg/hr	100 Units/100ml	1 Unit/ml	NSS	0.1-0.2#	Titrate
Isoproterenol HCl	Initiate: 5 mcg/min Range: 1-20 mcg/min	1mg/250ml [2mg/250ml]	0.004 mg/ml [0.008 mg/ml]	D5W or NSS	15-300 [7.5-150]	20 mcg/min
Labetalol HCl	Bolus: 20mg over 2 min then 40-80mg at 10 min intervals up to 300mg Infuse: 1-180 mg/hr	1000mg/200ml	5 mg/ml	D5W	0.2-36	Titrate
Lidocaine HCl	Bolus: 1mg/kg Infuse: 1-4 mg/min	2000mg/250ml	8 mg/ml	D5W or NSS	7.5-30	4 mg/min
Lorazepam	1-8 mg/hr	1mg/ml	1 mg/ml	D5W only	1-8	12 mg/hr
Midazolam HCl	1-8 mg/hr	1mg/ml	1 mg/ml	Undiluted	1-8	20 mg/hr
Milrinone Lactate	Bolus: 50 mcg/kg over 10 min Infuse: 0.375-0.75 mcg/kg/min (0.0225-0.045 mg/kg/hr)	20mg/100ml [100mg/250ml]	0.2 mg/ml [0.4 mg/ml]	D5W or NSS	0.1125-0.225# [0.056-0.1125]	1.13 mg/kg/day
Morphine Sulfate	1-10 mg/hr	100mg/100ml	1 mg/ml	D5W or NSS	1-10	Titrate
Naloxone HCl	Overdose: Bolus 0.4 mg Infuse: 0.25-6.25 mg/hr	2mg/500ml [10mg/100ml]	0.004 mg/ml [0.1 mg/ml]	D5W or NSS	62.5-1562.5 [2.5-62.5]	Titrate
Nicardipine HCl	Initiate: 5 mg/hr Range: 0.5-15 mg/hr	25mg/250ml	0.1 mg/ml	D5W or NSS	5-150	15 mg/hr
Nitroglycerin	5-250 mcg/min	50mg/250ml [150mg/250ml]	0.2 mg/ml [0.6 mg/ml]	D5W or NSS	1.5-75 [0.5-25]	Titrate
Norepinephrine Bitartrate	Initiate: 8-12 mcg/min Maintenance: 2-4 mcg/min	1mg/250ml [32mg/250ml]	0.004 mg/ml [0.128 mg/ml]	D5W or NSS	30-180 [0.94-1.88]	20 mcg/min
Octreotide Acetate	25-50 mcg/hr	500mcg/500ml [1000mcg/250ml]	1 mcg/ml [4 mcg/ml]	D5W or NSS	25-50 [6.25-12.5]	Titrate

138

16b: Infusions Commonly Used in the ICU (continued)

DRUG	USUAL DOSE	STANDARD DILUTION [concentrated dilution]	STANDARD CONCENTRATION [concentrated]	SOLUTION	RATE (ml/hr) (ml/kg/hr)[a] [concentrated]	MAXIMUM DOSE
Pancuronium Bromide	Bolus: 0.04-0.1 mg/kg over 1-2 min Infuse: 0.05 mg/kg/hr	20mg/250ml [40mg/250ml]	0.08mg/ml [0.16 mg/ml]	D5W or NSS	*0.625[a]* *[0.3125]*	Titrate
Pentobarbital Sodium	50 mg/min	2500mg/500ml	5 mg/ml	NSS	600	Titrate
Phenylephrine HCl	Initiate: 100-180 mcg/min Maintain: 40-60 mcg/min	10mg/500ml [60mg/250ml]	0.02mg/ml [0.24 mg/ml]	D5W or NSS	120-540 [10-45]	Titrate
Phenytoin Sodium	Bolus: 15-20 mg/kg Infuse 25-50 mg/min	1000mg/250ml	4 mg/ml	NSS only	375-750	50 mg/min
Procainamide HCl	Bolus: 17 mg/kg over 1 hour Infuse Maintenance: 1-4 mg/min	2000mg/250ml [2000mg/100ml]	8 mg/ml [20 mg/ml]	D5W or NSS	7.5-30 [3-12]	6 mg/min (50 mg/kg/d)
Propofol	5-50 mcg/kg/min (0.3-3 mg/kg/hr)	1000mg/100ml	10 mg/ml	Premix	*0.03-0.3[#]*	Titrate
Prostaglandin E1	0.2-0.6 mcg/kg/hr	500mcg/250ml	2 mcg/ml	D5W	*0.1-0.3[#]*	Titrate
Ranitidine HCl	6.25 mg/hr	150mg/150ml	1 mg/ml	D5W or NSS	6.25	400 mg/day
Sodium Nitroprusside	0.3-10 mcg/kg/min (0.018-0.6 mg/kg/hr)	50mg/250ml [150mg/250ml]	0.2 mg/ml [0.6 mg/ml]	D5W	*0.09-3[#]* *[0.03-1]*	10 mcg/kg/min
Tacrolimus	0.05-0.1 mg/kg/day over 24 hours	0.004-0.02mg/ml	Varies	D5W or NSS	Varies	Varies
Trimethaphan Camsylate	0.3-6 mg/min	500mg/500ml	1 mg/ml	D5W or NSS	18-360	10 mg/min
Urokinase	Pulmonary embolism (PE): Bolus: 4,400 IU/kg Infuse: 4,400 IU/kg/hr for 12 hr Coronary Artery Thrombus (CAT): Bolus: 2,500-10,000 IU Infuse: 6,000 IU/min	PE: 2,000,000 IU/500ml CAT: 500,000 IU/250ml	PE: 4,000 IU/ml CAT: 2,000 IU/ml	D5W or NSS	*PE: 1.1[#]* CAT: 180	Varies
Vasopressin	0.1-0.4 Units/min	250 Units/250ml	1 Unit/ml	D5W	6-24	0.6 Units/min
Vecuronium Bromide	Bolus: 0.08-0.1 mg/kg Infuse: 0.05-0.1 mg/kg/hr	20mg/100ml [100mg/100ml]	0.2 mg/ml [1 mg/ml]	D5W or NSS	*0.25-0.5[#]* *[0.05-0.1]*	Titrate
Verapamil HCl	5-10 mg/hr	40mg/100ml	0.4 mg/ml	D5W or NSS	12.5-25	10 mg/hr

16c: Rate Calculation (ml/hr) for Weight Based Dosing Regimens

Dose (ml/kg/hr)	Patient Weight					
	50 kg	60 kg	70 kg	80 kg	90 kg	100 kg
0.0047	0.235 ml/hr	0.282 ml/hr	0.329 ml/hr	0.376 ml/hr	0.423 ml/hr	0.47 ml/hr
0.03	1.5 ml/hr	1.8 ml/hr	2.1 ml/hr	2.4 ml/hr	2.7 ml/hr	3 ml/hr
0.0375	1.875 ml/hr	2.25 ml/hr	2.625 ml/hr	3 ml/hr	3.375 ml/hr	3.75 ml/hr
0.05	2.5 ml/hr	3 ml/hr	3.5 ml/hr	4 ml/hr	4.5 ml/hr	5 ml/hr
0.05625	2.8125 ml/hr	3.375 ml/hr	3.9375 ml/hr	4.5 ml/hr	5.0625 ml/hr	5.625 ml/hr
0.075	3.75 ml/hr	4.5 ml/hr	5.25 ml/hr	6 ml/hr	6.75 ml/hr	7.5 ml/hr
0.09	4.5 ml/hr	5.4 ml/hr	6.3 ml/hr	7.2 ml/hr	8.1 ml/hr	9 ml/hr
0.09375	4.69 ml/hr	5.6275 ml/hr	6.565 ml/hr	7.5 ml/hr	8.44 ml/hr	9.375 ml/hr
0.1	5 ml/hr	6 ml/hr	7 ml/hr	8 ml/hr	9 ml/hr	10 ml/hr
0.1125	5.625 ml/hr	6.75 ml/hr	7.875 ml/hr	9 ml/hr	10.125 ml/hr	11.25 ml/hr
0.15	7.5 ml/hr	9 ml/hr	10.5 ml/hr	12 ml/hr	13.5 ml/hr	15 ml/hr
0.2	10 ml/hr	12 ml/hr	14 ml/hr	16 ml/hr	18 ml/hr	20 ml/hr
0.225	11.25 ml/hr	13.5 ml/hr	15.75 ml/hr	18 ml/hr	20.25 ml/hr	22.5 ml/hr
0.25	12.5 ml/hr	15 ml/hr	17.5 ml/hr	20 ml/hr	22.5 ml/hr	25 ml/hr
0.3	15 ml/hr	18 ml/hr	21 ml/hr	24 ml/hr	27 ml/hr	30 ml/hr
0.3125	15.625 ml/hr	18.75 ml/hr	21.875 ml/hr	25 ml/hr	28.125 ml/hr	31.25 ml/hr
0.5	25 ml/hr	30 ml/hr	35 ml/hr	40 ml/hr	45 ml/hr	50 ml/hr
0.6	30 ml/hr	36 ml/hr	42 ml/hr	48 ml/hr	54 ml/hr	60 ml/hr
0.625	31.25 ml/hr	37.5 ml/hr	43.75 ml/hr	50 ml/hr	56.25 ml/hr	62.5 ml/hr
0.75	37.5 ml/hr	45 ml/hr	52.5 ml/hr	60 ml/hr	67.5 ml/hr	75 ml/hr
1	50 ml/hr	60 ml/hr	70 ml/hr	80 ml/hr	90 ml/hr	100 ml/hr
1.1	55 ml/hr	66 ml/hr	77 ml/hr	88 ml/hr	99 ml/hr	110 ml/hr
1.2	60 ml/hr	72 ml/hr	84 ml/hr	96 ml/hr	108 ml/hr	120 ml/hr
3	150 ml/hr	180 ml/hr	210 ml/hr	240 ml/hr	270 ml/hr	300 ml/hr

Anderson PO, Knoben JE. Handbook of Clinical Drug Data, 8th ed. Appleton & Lange, Stamford, 1997
McEvoy GK. AHFS Drug Information. American Society of Health-System Pharmacists, Bethesda, 1998
Trissel LA. Handbook on Injectable Drugs, 9th ed. American Society of Health-System Pharmacists, Bethesda,1996

16d: Therapeutic Drug Monitoring Guidelines for Selected Agents

Drug	Half-life (h)	Therapeutic Range	Potentially Toxic Range	Time to Steady-state[1]	When to Sample[2]
Aminoglycosides	Normal: 2-3h; Anephric: 30-60h	Gentamicin, Tobramycin, and Netilmicin[3]: peak 4-8 mg/L; trough<2 mg/L. Amikacin[3]: peak 20-30 mg/L; trough<10 mg/L.	Gentamicin, Tobramycin, Netilmicin[3]: peak>10 mg/L; trough>2 mg/L; Amikacin[3]: peak>30 mg/L; trough>10 mg/L	Normal: 12-24 h; Anephric: 6-12 d	Obtain peak and trough levels
Carbamazepine	15-20 h	4-12 mg/L	>12 mg/L	60-80 h	Trough
Chloramphenicol	4 h	Peak 15-25 mg/L; Trough 5-10 mg/L	Peak > 25 mg/L; Trough > 10 mg/L	18 h	Obtain peak 1 hour after the end of infusion
Cyclosporine	16-26h	100-400 µg/L	>400 µg/L	80-130h	IV: after 4 days of continuous IV therapy PO: trough level
Digoxin	24-36 h	CHF: 0.6-1.2 µg/L (0.7-1.4µmol/L); SVT: 0.6-2.0 µg/L (0.7-2.4µmol/L)	> 2.0 µg/L (>2.4µmol/L)	5-7 d	At least 12 h after dose given
Ethosuximide	30-50 h	40-100 mg/L	> 100 mg/L	180-250 h	Trough
5-flucytosine	4 h	35-70 mg/L	> 100 mg/L	20 h	Trough
Lidocaine	Normal: 1h; CHF: 4-6 h; CLD*: 6h	2-6 mg/L (6-21.5 µmol/L)	> 6 mg/L (> 21.5µmol/L)	6-24 h	At least 6h after start of infusion
Lithium	20 h	0.8-1.2 mEq/L	>1.5 mEq/L	100 h	Morning trough
Phenobarbital	5 d	10-30 mg/L	> 35 mg/L	20-30 d	Obtain trough at least 2-3 weeks after initiation of therapy or change in dose[6]
Phenytoin	75-125 h	10-20 mg/L (40-80 µmol/L)	>25 mg/L (>100 µmol/L)	7-14 d	Obtain trough at least 5-7 days after initiation or change in dose[6]
Phenytoin, free	75-125 h	1-2 mg/L (4-8 µmol/L)	>2.5 mg/L (>10 µmol/L)	7-14 d	Obtain only in patients with altered protein binding, e.g., renal failure, hepatic failure, malnutrition
Primidone	7 h	8-12 mg/L	>12 mg/L	35 h	Obtain trough level for primidone; also obtain trough level for phenobarbital (metabolite) 2-3 weeks after initiation of therapy or change in dose
Procainamide	P*: 3 h; NAPA: 6h	4-10 mg/L (P* only) (17-42.5 µmol/L)	>10 mg/L (P* only >42.5 µmol/L); >30 mg/L (P*+NAPA >127.5 µmol/L)	P*: 15 h; NAPA: 30h	IV: Sample 12h after initiation PO: Trough
Quinidine	6.5 h	2-5 mg/L (4.6-11.5 µmol/L)	>10 mg/L (>23 µmol/L)	30 h	Trough
Tacrolimus	15 h	5-8 ng/mL	>10 ng/mL	75 h	Trough
Theophylline	8.3 h	5-15 mg/L (27.5-85 µmol/L)	>20 mg/L	36-48 h	IV: anytime during the infusion PO: trough level
Valproic acid	6-12 h	50-100 mg/L	>100 mg/L	35-60 h	Trough
Vancomycin	Normal: 7 h; Anephric: 7 days	Peak: 30-50 mg/L; Trough: 5-15 mg/L	Peak: >60 mg/L; Trough: >20 mg/L	Normal: 30 h; Anephric: 14-28 d	Obtain peak and trough levels

Steady-state assumes stable physiologic status; [a]Obtain trough level just before the next dose. Obtain peak level one hour after end of infusion. *Higher peak levels may be necessary for more serious infections; [c]Chronic liver disease ; [d]Procainamide, [e]Trough levels may be obtained more frequently in patients with acute illness (e.g. status epilepticus) in whom therapeutic levels need to be established quickly.

1. Evans WE, Schentag JJ, Jusko WJ, eds. Applied Pharmacokietics, 3rd ed. Vancouver, WA: Applied Therapeutics, Inc., 1992.
2. Winter ME, ed. Basic Clinical Pharmacokinetics, 2nd ed. Vancouver, WA: Applied Therapeutics, Inc., 1988

16e: Calculating IV Drips in Your Head

The formula to compute any drip can be expressed by the following formula:

(A) Concentration (mcg/cc) X drip rate (#cc/min) = dose (mcg/min)

<u>STEP 1</u>: Determine the concentration of the drip in mcg per cc.

Find out how the nurse mixed the drip. For IV NTG it may be 50mg in 250cc of D5W. Dopamine may be 400 mg in 500cc D5W. This mixture can be thought of as a fraction:

50mg/250cc NTG or 400mg/500cc Dopamine

You want to convert this fraction to one with a denominator of 1000. For IV NTG multiply by 4/4. For the dopamine multiply by 2/2.

50mg/250cc x 4/4 = 200mg/1000cc
400mg/500cc x 2/2 = 800mg/1000cc

To convert this new fraction to mcg/cc is easy. We simply divide both numerator and denominator by 1000. In the numerator division by 1000 changes mg to mcg. In the denominator division by 1000 changes 1000cc to 1cc.
Note that when we divide the numerator and denominator by 1000 the numbers stay the same, only the units change:

200mg/1000cc = 200mcg/cc
800mg/1000cc = 800mcg/cc

<u>STEP 2</u>: Determine the total number of mcg/min needed.

For drips like IV NTG this is simply the MD's order: Start IV NTG at 20mcg/min.
For 'per kilo' drips like dopamine the number of mcg/min is the product of the pt's mass in kilograms times the rate:

mcg/min = mcg/kg/min x #kg

Example: Determine the mcg/min for a 193 LB pt ordered to get 5 mcg/kg/min of dopamine.

First use the <u>CONVERTING POUNDS TO KILOGRAMS</u> technique to determine that 193 lbs = 88 kg.
Next multiply 88 kg by 5 mcg/kg/min to determine the mcg/min:

mcg/min = 5 mcg/kg/min x 88 kg
        = 440 mcg/min.

<u>STEP 3</u>: Determine the drip rate.

From STEP1 we know the concentration of the drip in mcg/cc. From STEP2 we know the how many mcg/min of drug we want to administer. In STEP 3 we will determine the drip rate (cc/min). This will complete formula (A):

concentration (mcg/cc) x drip rate (#cc/min) = dose (mcg/min)

Usually drip rates are expressed as cc/hr as in IV NTG at 20cc/hr. To convert cc/hr to cc/min simply replace hr by 60min. Formula (A) now becomes:

concentration (mcg/cc) x drip rate (#cc/60 min) = dose (mcg/min)

To determine the drip rate we need to pick a number for cc/min. Keep in mind the following relationships:

6/60 = 0.1	12/60 = 0.2	15/60 = 0.25
20/60 = one third 30/60 = 0.5	45/60 = three quarters	
40/60 = two thirds 60/60 = 1.0		

First pick a number that gets you close to the desired value. Then modify it for precision.
Let's return to the example of the 193 LB patient to be placed on 5 mcg/kg/min of dopamine. Dopamine is mixed 400 mg/500 cc.

<u>STEP 1</u>: Concentration

400 mg/500cc x 2/2 = 800 mg/1000cc
dividing by 1000/1000   = 800 mcg/cc.

<u>STEP 2:</u> Number of mcg/min = 440 mcg/min   (see example above)

<u>STEP 3:</u> Determine the drip rate.

Formula (A) becomes:

800 mcg/cc x #cc/60 min = 440 mcg/min

If we choose 30cc/60 min we obtain:

800 mcg/cc x 30cc/60 min = 800 mcg/min x 0.5
                          = 400 mcg/min

Thus at drip rate of 30cc/60min we will deliver 400 mcg/min of dopamine. This is close to but not quite our desired dose. Here's where you need to be clever. If 30cc/60min delivers 400 mcg/min then 3cc/60min (3 is one tenth of 30) will deliver 40mcg/min (40 is one tenth of 400). Thus a drip rate of 33cc/60min will deliver the desired dose of 440 mcg/min.

Clinical disorder or indication	Recommended Therapy (options)		
Stroke prevention after transient ischemic attack or stroke (see *Acute stroke* for treatment during event)	Aspirin 75-1,300 mg/day (Aspirin plus clopidogrel 75 mg qd) (Aspirin plus ticlopine 250 mg BID) (Clopidogrel 75 mg qd or Ticlopidine 250 mg BID if aspirin fails or contraindicated) (Warfarin, INR 2-3 if aspirin failure or contraindication)		
Asymptomatic carotid stenosis	Aspirin 325 mg/day (Aspirin 75-1,300 mg/day)		
Atrial fibrillation **Risk factors:** prior TIA, stroke, systemic embolism, hypertension, CHF, rheumatic mitral valve disease, prosthetic heart valve	Age	Risk factors	Recommendation
	< 65 years	Absent	Aspirin 325 mg qd
		Present	Warfarin, INR 2.0-3.0 (target 2.5)
	65-75 years	Absent	Aspirin or warfarin
		Present	Warfarin, INR 2.0-3.0 (target 2.5)
	> 75 years	All patients	Warfarin INR 2.0-3.0 (target 2.5)
Atrial fibrillation: Elective cardioversion	> 2 days AF: Warfarin, INR 2.0-3.0 X 3 weeks prior to cardioversion. Continue anticoagulation after cardioversion until in sinus rhythm for 4 weeks. < 2 days of SVT or AF: No therapy		
Stable angina / coronary artery disease	Aspirin 160-325 mg/day		
Unstable angina	ASA 160-325 mg/d or Ticlopidine 250 mg bid if ASA intolerant If hospitalized, start heparin 75 U/kg bolus, then 1,250 U/h, adjust to APTT 1.5-2.0 X control for 3-4 days or until syndrome resolves		
Deep venous thrombosis	• Heparin: 5-10,000 load, then 1,300 U/H, check and adjust Q6H until APTT 1.5-2.5 X control. Continue 4-7 days with warfarin, INR 2.0-3.0 or • Low molecular weight heparin (e.g. Enoxaparin 1 mg/kg SC q12h, others may be approved for this indication by publication) • Warfarin: Start with heparin or enoxaparin therapy at 5-10 mg, then adjust daily to INR 2.0-3.0 X 3 - 6 months, or long term if continued risk Thrombolytic Rx (when indicated, choose one regimen): • Streptokinase: 250,000 IU load, then 100,000 IU/h X 48-72H • Urokinase: 4,400 IU/kg load, then 4,400 IU/kg/h X 24-48H • rtPA: 100 mg infused over 2 H Restart heparin without a load once APTT or TT < 1.5 X control		
Pulmonary embolism	• Heparin: load and maintenance as for deep venous thrombosis. • Warfarin: Start with heparin therapy at 5-10 mg, then adjust daily to INR 2.0-3.0 X 6 mos Thrombolytic Rx (when indicated, choose one regimen): • Streptokinase: 250,000 IU load, then 100,000 IU/h X 24 H • Urokinase: 4,400 IU/kg load, then 4,400 IU/kg/h X 12 H • rtPA: 100 mg infused over 2 H Restart heparin without a load once APTT or TT < 1.5 X control		
Rheumatic mitral valve disease	Systemic embolism or a fib: Warfarin, INR 2.0-3.0, target 2.5 Left atrial diameter > 5.5 cm: Warfarin, INR 2.0-3.0, target 2.5 Add aspirin (80-100 mg/d), clopidogrel 75 mg qd, or ticlopidine 250 bid if warfarin failure		
Mitral annular calcification	Systemic embolism hx or associated atrial fibrillation: Warfarin INR 2.0-3.0 Not recommended if no h/o embolism or a-fib		
Mitral valve prolapse	Not recommended if no h/o systemic embolism, TIAs or a fib Unexplained TIAs: Aspirin 160-325 mg/d Systemic embolism, a fib, or recurrent TIAs despite ASA: Warfarin INR 2.0-3.0		
Patent foramen ovale or Atrial septal defect	Asymptomatic: Not recommended Unexplained TIAs, venous thrombosis, pulmonary/systemic embolism: Warfarin INR 2.0-3.0 (unless venous interruption or closure of PFO is considered preferable)		
Bioprosthetic mitral valve/sinus rhythm	Mitral, sinus rhythm: Warfarin, INR 2.0-3.0 X 3 mos post op; Aspirin 162 mg/d long term Aortic, sinus rhythm: Warfarin; INR 2.0 – 3.0 X 3 mos optional; ASA 162 mg/d long term With a fib or systemic embolization: Warfarin INR 2.0 – 3.0 long term		
Prosthetic heart valves	Bileaflet aortic, normal L atrium, EF, and sinus rhythm: Warfarin, INR 2.0 – 3.0 (target 2.5) Tilting disk, bileaflet mitral valve, or bileaflet aortic with a fib: Warfarin 2.5-3.5 (target 3.0) (Tilting disk, any bileaflet plus a fib: Warfarin 2.0-3.0 (target 2.5) plus aspirin 80-100 mg/d) Caged ball or caged disk: Warfarin 2.5-3.5 (target 3.0) plus aspirin 80-100 mg/d Any valve plus additional risk factor: Warfarin 2.5-3.5 (target 3.0) plus aspirin 80-100 mg/d		
Myocardial infarction (see *Acute Myocardial infarction* for indications)	Heparin: load and maintenance as for deep venous thrombosis Streptokinase 1,500,000 U IV over 1 H or APSAC 30 U IV over 5 minutes or rtPA: 15 mg IV bolus, then 0.75 mg/kg (but not > 50 mg) over 30 minutes, then 0.5 mg/kg (but not > 35 mg) over 60 minutes.		

Note: Warfarin should not be during pregnancy. Heparin should be given during pregnancy when antithrombotic therapy is indicated.

Fifth ACCP consensus conference on antithrombotic therapy. Chest 114(suppl): 439S - 769S, 1998

17a: Antiretroviral Therapy in HIV Disease[1]

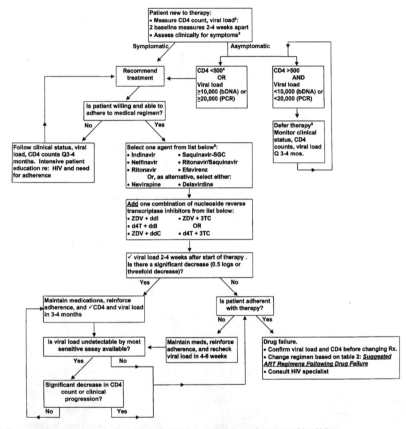

Patient new to therapy:
- Measure CD4 count, viral load[2]:
- 2 baseline measures 2-4 weeks apart
- Assess clinically for symptoms[3]

Symptomatic / Asymptomatic

Recommend treatment

CD4 <500[4]
OR
Viral load
≥10,000 (bDNA) or
≥20,000 (PCR)

CD4 >500
AND
Viral load
<10,000 (bDNA) or
<20,000 (PCR)

Is patient willing and able to adhere to medical regimen?

No / Yes

Defer therapy[5]
Monitor clinical status, CD4 counts, viral load Q 3-4 mos.

Follow clinical status, viral load, CD4 counts Q3-4 months. Intensive patient education re: HIV and need for adherence

Select one agent from list below[6]:
- Indinavir • Saquinavir-SGC
- Nelfinavir • Ritonavir/Saquinavir
- Ritonavir • Efavirenz
Or, as alternative, select either:
- Nevirapine • Delavirdine

Add one combination of nucleoside reverse transcriptase inhibitors from list below:
- ZDV + ddI • ZDV + 3TC
- d4T + ddI OR
- ZDV + ddC • d4T + 3TC

✓ viral load 2-4 weeks after start of therapy . Is there a significant decrease (0.5 logs or threefold decrease)?

Yes / No

Maintain medications, reinforce adherence, and ✓CD4 and viral load in 3-4 months

Is patient adherent with therapy?

No / Yes

Is viral load undetectable by most sensitive assay available?

Yes / No

Maintain meds, reinforce adherence, and recheck viral load in 4-6 weeks

Drug failure.
- Confirm viral load and CD4 before changing Rx.
- Change regimen based on table 2: *Suggested ART Regimens Following Drug Failure*
- Consult HIV specialist

Significant decrease in CD4 count or clinical progression?

No / Yes

1. Recommendations change frequently. Check www.hivatis.org and www.pocketdoctor.com for most up to date guidelines.
2. Viral load should not be measured for four weeks after intercurrent infection/illness or immunization.
3. Thrush, unexplained fever, and those diagnosed with AIDS.
4. Controversial. Some experts advocate withholding therapy in asymptomatic patients with stable CD4 350-500 cells/mm³ and viral loads <10,000 (bDNA) or <20,000 (PCR).
5. Controversial. Some experts advocate treatment in this situation.
ZDV = zidovudine; ddI = didanosine; ddC = zalcitabine; d4T = stavudine; 3TC = lamivudine. See table 1, *Antiretroviral agents* for dosages.
6. Abacavir and amprenavir may be added to this list shortly.

Centers for Disease Control and Prevention. Report of the NIH Panel to define principles of therapy of HIV infection and guidelines for the use of antiretroviral agents in HIV-infected adults and adolescents. HIV/AIDS Treatment Information Service, 12/1/98, www.hivatis.org.

17b: Antiretroviral Agents

Protease Inhibitors

Drug	Dose (oral)	Considerations	Common side effects
Indinavir (Crixivan)	800mg po q 8hr	taken 1 hr before or 2 hrs after a meal increase po fluids	nausea, abdominal pain, headache diarrhea, vomiting, nephrolithiasis, increased indirect bilirubin
Nelfinavir (Viracept)	750mg po tid	taken with food	nausea, flatulence, nausea, rash
Ritonavir (Norvir)	600mg po q12h	taken with food Start with 200 mg q12h and gradually increase over 5-7 days to 600 q12h	nausea, diarrhea, vomiting, taste perversion, abdominal pain, circumoral paresthesia, increased triglycerides
Saquinavir HGC (Invirase)	600mg po tid	taken with a meal	diarrhea, nausea, abdominal pain, headache
Saquinavir SGC (Fortovase)	1200mg po tid	taken with a meal or up to 2hrs after	diarrhea, nausea, abdominal pain, dyspepsia, headache
Ritonavir + Saquinavir Combination	400mg po bid 400 mg po bid	Dose same - HGC or SGC; taken with food	As noted above
Amprenavir (Agenerase)	1200 mg po bid	awaiting FDA approval	rash, diarrhea, headache, nausea

Nucleoside Reverse Transciptase Inhibitors (NRTI)

Drug	Dose (oral)	Considerations	Common side effects
Zidovudine(Retrovir, ZDV)	300mg bid or 200mg tid		anemia, neutropenia, GI intolerance, headache, insomnia, asthenia
Didanosine, (Videx, ddI)	>60kg: 200mg bid, <60kg: 125mg bid	take on empty stomach	pancreatitis, peripheral neuropathy, nausea, diarrhea
Zalcitabine, (HIVID, ddC)	0.75mg tid		peripheral neuropathy, stomatitis
Stavudine(Zerit, d4T)	>60kg: 40mg bid, <60kg: 30mg bid		peripheral neuropathy
Lamivudine, (Epivir, 3TC)	150mg bid <50kg: 2mg/kg bid		adverse effects uncommon, rarely headache, GI intolerance
Abacavir (Ziagen)	300 mg po bid	3% of patients develop hypersensitivity reaction with fever, malaise, nausea, occasional rash. Resolves w/n 2 days of stopping medication. Do not rechallenge, has been associated with death. Read package insert..	Headache, nausea

Non-Nucleoside Reverse Transcriptase Inhibitors (NNRTI)*

Drug	Dose (oral)	Considerations	Common side effects
Nevirapine (Viramune)	200mg bid	Start with 200mg qd for first 14 days	rash, increased transaminases, hepatitis
Delavirdine(Rescriptor)	400mg tid		rash, headaches
Efavirenz (Sustiva)	600 mg po qd	Usually dosed qhs due to initial side effects. False positive cannibold test	Initial dizziness, lightheadedness, insomnia, rash

Suggested ART Regimens Following Drug Failure
(see table1 for specifics of drug classes, drugs)

Failed regimen	Possible new regimens	
Nelfinavir + 2 NRTIs	2 New NRTIs plus	Ritonavir, or Indinavir, or Ritonavir/Saquinavir, or Ritonavir + 1 NNRTI , or Indinavir + 1 NNRTI
Ritonavir + 2 NRTIs or Indinavir + 2NRTIs	2 new NRTIs plus	Ritonavir/Saquinavir, or Nelfinavir + 1 NNRTI , or Nelfinavir/Saquinavir
Saquinavir + 2 NRTIs	2 new NRTIs plus	Ritonavir/Saquinavir, or Indinavir + 1 NNRTI
2 NRTIs + NNRTI	2 new NRTIs plus	1 protease inhibitor
2 NRTIs	2 new NRTIs plus	1 protease inhibitor , or Ritonavir/saquinavir, or
	1 new NRTI plus	1 NNRTI + 1 protease inhibitor, or
	1 NNRTI plus	2 protease inhibitors
1 NRTI	2 new NRTIs plus	1 protease inhibitor, or 1 NNRTI, or
	1 new NRTI plus	1 NNRTI + 1 protease inhibitor

17c: Prophylactic Therapies for HIV Infection

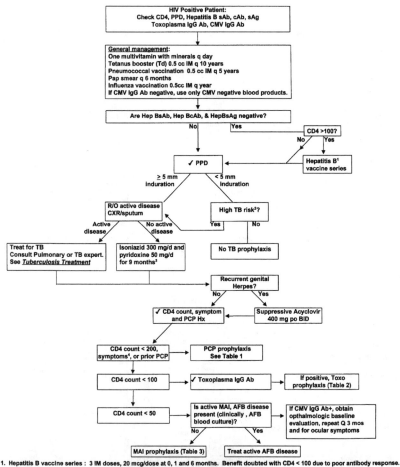

HIV Positive Patient:
Check CD4, PPD, Hepatitis B sAb, cAb, sAg
Toxoplasma IgG Ab, CMV IgG Ab

General management:
One multivitamin with minerals q day
Tetanus booster (Td) 0.5 cc IM q 10 years
Pneumococcal vaccination 0.5 cc IM q 5 years
Pap smear q 6 months
Influenza vaccination 0.5cc IM q year
If CMV IgG Ab negative, use only CMV negative blood products.

Are Hep BsAb, Hep BcAB, & HepBsAg negative?
No / Yes

CD4 >100?
No / Yes

Hepatitis B[1] vaccine series

✓ PPD
≥ 5 mm induration / < 5 mm induration

R/O active disease CXR/sputum
Active disease / No active disease

High TB risk[2]?
Yes / No

Treat for TB Consult Pulmonary or TB expert. *See Tuberculosis Treatment*

Isoniazid 300 mg/d and pyridoxine 50 mg/d for 9 months[3]

No TB prophylaxis

Recurrent genital Herpes?
No / Yes

✓ CD4 count, symptom and PCP Hx

Suppressive Acyclovir 400 mg po BID

CD4 count < 200, symptoms[4], or prior PCP

PCP prophylaxis See Table 1

CD4 count < 100

✓ Toxoplasma IgG Ab

If positive, Toxo prophylaxis (Table 2)

CD4 count < 50

Is active MAI, AFB disease present (clinically, AFB blood culture)?
No / Yes

If CMV IgG Ab+, obtain opthalmologic baseline evaluation, repeat Q 3 mos and for ocular symptoms

MAI prophylaxis (Table 3)

Treat active AFB disease

1. Hepatitis B vaccine series : 3 IM doses, 20 mcg/dose at 0, 1 and 6 months. Benefit doubted with CD4 < 100 due to poor antibody response.
2. High risk: exposure to TB, Injection drug user, homeless persons, and migrant workers.
3. Requires monthly clinical monitoring and liver transaminases at 1 and 3 months; alternative short course regimens are available.
4. Recurrent mucosal candidiasis, unexplained fevers ≥ 2 weeks

Centers for Disease Control and Prevention. 1997 USPHS/IDSA guidelines for the prevention of opportunistic infections in persons infected with human immunodeficiency virus. MMWR 46 (No. RR-12), 1997
Centers for Disease Control and Prevention. Prevention and treatment of tuberculosis among patients infected with human immunodeficiency virus: principles of therapy and revised recommendations. MMWR 47 (No. RR-20), 1998

17d: HIV Post-Exposure Prophylaxis (PEP)[1]

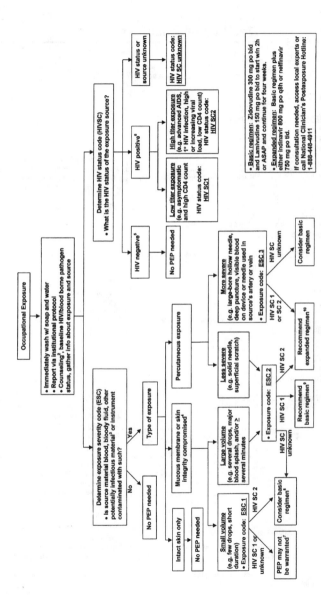

Occupational Exposure
- Immediately wash w/ soap and water
- Report via institutional protocol
- Counseling[2], baseline HIV/blood borne pathogen status, gather info about exposure and source

Determine exposure severity code (ESC)
- Is source material blood, bloody fluid, other potentially infectious material[3] or instrument contaminated with such?

Yes → Type of exposure
No → No PEP needed

Type of exposure:
- Mucous membrane or skin integrity compromised[4]
- Percutaneous exposure

Mucous membrane or skin integrity compromised[4]:
- Small volume (e.g. few drops, short duration) — Exposure code: **ESC 1**
  - HIV SC 1 or unknown → PEP may not be warranted[7]
  - HIV SC 2 → Consider basic regimen[8]
- Large volume (e.g. several drops, major blood splash, and/or ≥ several minutes)
  - HIV SC unknown
  - HIV SC 1 → Recommend basic regimen[9]
  - HIV SC 2 →

Percutaneous exposure:
- Less severe (e.g. solid needle, superficial scratch) — Exposure code: **ESC 2**
  - HIV SC 1
  - HIV SC 2
- More severe (e.g. large-bore hollow needle, deep puncture, visible blood on device or needle used in source's artery or vein) — Exposure code: **ESC 3**
  - HIV SC 1 or SC 2 → Recommend expanded regimen[10]
  - HIV SC unknown → Consider basic regimen

Determine HIV status code (HIVSC)
- What is the HIV status of the exposure source?

- **HIV negative[5]** → No PEP needed
- **HIV positive[6]**
  - Low titer exposure (e.g. asymptomatic and high CD4 count) HIV status code: **HIV SC1**
  - High titer exposure (e.g. advanced AIDS, 1° HIV infection, high or increasing viral load, low CD4 count) HIV status code: **HIV SG2**
- **HIV status or source unknown** → HIV status code: **HIV SC unknown**

- **Basic regimen:** Zidovudine 300 mg po bid and Lamivudine 150 mg po bid to start w/in 2h or ASAP and continue for four weeks.
- **Expanded regimen:** Basic regimen plus either Indinavir 800 mg po q8h or nelfinavir 750 mg po tid.

If consultation needed, access local experts or call National Clinician's Postexposure Hotline: 1-888-448-4911

1. Adapted from and should be used in consultation with this reference: Centers for Disease Control and Prevention. Public Health Service Guidelines for the management of health care worker exposures to HIV and recommendations for post-exposure prophylaxis. MMWR 47 (No RR-7), 1998
2. Counseling to include: exposure risk, post exposure prophylaxis, safer sex methods, recommended precautions including avoidance of blood/organ donation, pregnancy and breast feeding.
3. Other potentially infectious material includes semen, vaginal secretions, cerebrospinal, synovial, pleural, peritoneal, pericardial or amniotic fluids; or tissue
4. Skin integrity compromised if chapped skin, dermatitis, abrasion, or open wound
5. Source considered HIV negative if negative HIV Ab, HIV by PCR, or HIV p24 Ag test performed at or near time of exposure and no evidence of recent retroviral-like illness.
6. Source considered HIV positive if positive lab test for HIV Ab, HIV by PCR, or HIV p24 Ag, or physician-diagnosed AIDS.
7. Exposure doesn't pose known risk for HIV transmission.
8. Negligible risk of transmission based on exposure. Whether risk of drug toxicity outweighs benefit of PEP decided by exposed health care worker (HCW) and clinician.
9. No risk of HIV transmission has been observed but PEP is appropriate. High HIV titer in source may justify PEP. Whether risk of drug toxicity outweighs benefit of PEP decided by exposed HCW and clinician.
10. Exposure indicates increased HIV transmission risk.

All listed in order of preference
All are given orally unless specified

Table 1: PCP prophylaxis

Drug	Dose	Side effects	Comments
TMP/SMX	1DS qd . 1SS qd 1DS tiw	Nausea, vomiting, pruritis, rash, cytopenias, fever, elevated transaminases	• Clearly drug of choice. • Many advocate desensitization for allergy . • Concomitant toxoplasmosis and bacterial prophylaxis.
Dapsone 100 mg qd		Rash, pruritis, hepatitis, anemia, neutropenia Hemolytic anemia w/wo G6PD deficiency	• Concomitant toxoplasmosis prophylaxis w/pyrimethamine 50 mg/wk & folinic acid 25 mg/wk. • Check G6PD deficiency before use.
Pentamidine, aerosolized	300 mg q month via Respigard II nebulizer	Cough, wheeze, laryngitis, chest pain, dyspnea	Associated with greater failure rate

Table 2: Toxoplasma prophylaxis - goal is to use one single regimen for PCP and toxo

Regimens	Dose	Side effects	Comments
TMP/SMX	1 DS qd 1 SS qd	see Table 1	• Regimen of choice. • Concomitant PCP prophylaxis.
Dapsone Pyrimethamine Leukovorin	50 mg qd 50 mg q wk 25 mg q wk	Marrow suppression, GI intolerance	Concomitant PCP prophylaxis.
Dapsone 200 mg q wk Pyrimethamine Leukovorin	75 mg q wk 25 mg q wk	see above and table 1	

Table 3: MAI prophylaxis

Drug	Dose	Side effects	Comments
Azithromycin	1200mg/wk	GI intolerance diarrhea	• Most cost-effective regimen • Break-through infections with little resistance.
Clarithromycin	500 mg bid	GI intolerance headache transaminase elevation	Break-through infections frequently resistant to macrolides
Rifabutin 300 mg qd		Orange urine, rash, GI intolerance, neutropenia dose related uveitis	• Avoid use with ritonavir and saquinavir, • Dose-reduced (halved) if used w/ crixivan, nelfinavir.

Abbreviations: PCP = pneumocystis carinii pneumonia; TMP/SMX = trimethoprim-sulfamethoxazole; DS = double strength; SS = single strength; toxo = toxoplasmosis; G6PD = glucose-6-phosphate dehydrogenase.

Centers for Disease Control and Prevention. 1997 USPHS/IDSA guidelines for the prevention of opportunistic infections in persons infected with human immunodeficiency virus. MMWR. 46(No. RR-12), 1997

18a: Acne

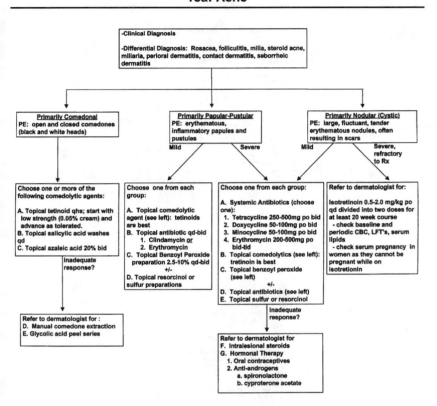

-Clinical Diagnosis

-Differential Diagnosis: Rosacea, folliculitis, milia, steroid acne, miliaria, perioral dermatitis, contact dermatitis, seborrheic dermatitis

Primarily Comedonal
PE: open and closed comedones (black and white heads)

Primarily Papular-Pustular
PE: erythematous, inflammatory papules and pustules

Mild — Severe

Primarily Nodular (Cystic)
PE: large, fluctuant, tender erythematous nodules, often resulting in scars

Mild — Severe, refractory to Rx

Choose one or more of the following comedolytic agents:

A. Topical tetinoid qhs; start with low strength (0.05% cream) and advance as tolerated.
B. Topical salicylic acid washes qd
C. Topical azaleic acid 20% bid

Inadequate response?

Refer to dermatologist for :
D. Manual comedone extraction
E. Glycolic acid peel series

Choose one from each group:

A. Topical comedolytic agent (see left): tetinoids are best
B. Topical antibiotic qd-bid
   1. Clindamycin or
   2. Erythromycin
C. Topical Benzoyl Peroxide preparation 2.5-10% qd-bid
   +/-
D. Topical resorcinol or sulfur preparations

Choose one from each group:

A. Systemic Antibiotics (choose one):
   1. Tetracycline 250-500mg po bid
   2. Doxycycline 50-100mg po bid
   3. Minocycline 50-100mg po bid
   4. Erythromycin 200-500mg po bid-tid
B. Topical comedolytics (see left): tretinoin is best
C. Topical benzoyl peroxide (see left)
   +/-
D. Topical antibiotics (see left)
E. Topical sulfur or resorcinol

Inadequate response?

Refer to dermatologist for
F. Intralesional steroids
G. Hormonal Therapy
   1. Oral contraceptives
   2. Anti-androgens
      a. spironolactone
      b. cyproterone acetate

Refer to dermatologist for:

Isotretinoin 0.5-2.0 mg/kg po qd divided into two doses for at least 20 week course
   - check baseline and periodic CBC, LFT's, serum lipids
   - check serum pregnancy in women as they cannot be pregnant while on isotretionin

Berger, TG et al. Manual of Therapy for Skin Diseases. New York: Churchill Livingstone, 1990.
Leyden, J and Shalita, A. Rational Therapy for Acne Vulgaris: and Update on Topical Treatment. J Am Acad Dermatol 1986; 15:907-15.
Plewing, G and Kligman, AM. Acne and Rosacea. New York: Springer Verlag, 1993.
Shalita A. Topical Acne Therapy. Dermatol Clin 1983;1:399-403.

18b: Psoriasis

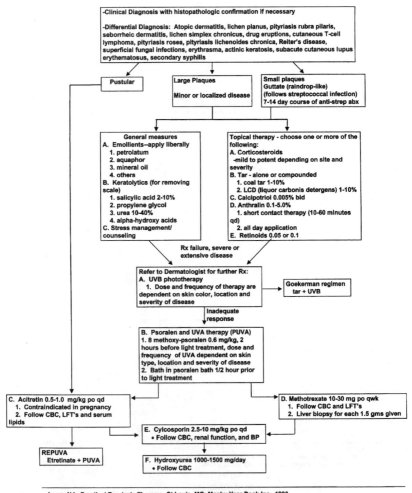

-Clinical Diagnosis with histopathologic confirmation if necessary

-Differential Diagnosis: Atopic dermatitis, lichen planus, pityriasis rubra pilaris, seborrheic dermatitis, lichen simplex chronicus, drug eruptions, cutaneous T-cell lymphoma, pityriasis rosea, pityriasis lichenoides chronica, Reiter's disease, superficial fungal infections, erythrasma, actinic keratosis, subacute cutaneous lupus erythematosus, secondary syphilis

Pustular

Large Plaques

Minor or localized disease

Small plaques
Guttate (raindrop-like)
(follows streptococcal infection)
7-14 day course of anti-strep abx

General measures
A. Emollients—apply liberally
  1. petrolatum
  2. aquaphor
  3. mineral oil
  4. others
B. Keratolytics (for removing scale)
  1. salicylic acid 2-10%
  2. propylene glycol
  3. urea 10-40%
  4. alpha-hydroxy acids
C. Stress management/counseling

Topical therapy - choose one or more of the following:
A. Corticosteroids
  -mild to potent depending on site and severity
B. Tar - alone or compounded
  1. coal tar 1-10%
  2. LCD (liquor carbonis detergens) 1-10%
C. Calcipotriol 0.005% bid
D. Anthralin 0.1-5.0%
  1. short contact therapy (10-60 minutes qd)
  2. all day application
E. Retinoids 0.05 or 0.1

Rx failure, severe or extensive disease

Refer to Dermatologist for further Rx:
A. UVB phototherapy
  1. Dose and frequency of therapy are dependent on skin color, location and severity of disease

Goekerman regimen
tar + UVB

Inadequate response

B. Psoralen and UVA therapy (PUVA)
1. 8 methoxy-psoralen 0.6 mg/kg, 2 hours before light treatment, dose and frequency of UVA dependent on skin type, location and severity of disease
2. Bath in psoralen bath 1/2 hour prior to light treatment

C. Acitretin 0.5-1.0 mg/kg po qd
  1. Contraindicated in pregnancy
  2. Follow CBC, LFT's and serum lipids

D. Methotrexate 10-30 mg po qwk
  1. Follow CBC and LFT's
  2. Liver biopsy for each 1.5 gms given

E. Cylcosporin 2.5-10 mg/kg po qd
• Follow CBC, renal function, and BP

REPUVA
Etretinate + PUVA

F. Hydroxyurea 1000-1500 mg/day
• Follow CBC

Lowe, NJ. Practical Psoriasis Therapy. St Louis, MO: Mosby Year Book Inc., 1993.
Marks, R. Topical Therapy for Psoriasis: General Principles. Dermatol Clin;2:382-8.
Weinstein, GD and Gottleib, AB. Therapy of Moderate-to-Severe Psoriasis. National Psoriasis Foundation. Portland, OR: Haber and Flora, Inc., 1993.

18c: Fungal Infection

A. Tinea Capitis	Choose one: a. Griseofulvin - 250mg po bid (microsized) or 125-187.5mg po bid (ultramicrosized) for 4-6 weeks b. Ketoconazole 200mg po qd (3.3mg/kg po qd in children) c. Itraconazole 100mg po qd for 6 weeks d. Fluconazole 50mg po qd for 10-20 days e. Terbenafine250mg po qd for 4-8 weeks

** treat affected family members and pets and dispose of contaminated combs, hats , etc.

B. Tinea Corporis and Cruris	1. Mild/localized cases a. topical imidazole or allylamine products (econazole, miconazole, terbinafine, naftifine, etc.)
	2. Severe/resistant cases (choose 1) a. Griseofulvin 125-187.5mg ultramicrosized po bid (250mg microsized) for 2-4 weeks b. Nizoral 200mg po qd for 3-6 weeks c. Itraconazole 100mg po qd for 15 days d. Fluconazole 150mg po qwk for 4 weeks e. Terbenafine 250mg po qd for 2-4 weeks

**drying powders such as Zeabsorb and aeration may facilitate treatment

C. Tinea Manum	Same as T. Corporis but may require longer duration and higher doses
D. Tinea Pedis	

E. Tinea Unguium (Onychomycosis)	1. Topical therapies are usually not effective. Choose 1 oral agent below:
	a. Terbinafine 250mg po qd for 6 weeks for fingernails, 12 weeks for toenails b. Itraconazole 200mg po qd for 12 weeks, or 200mg po bid for one week of each month for 3-6 months c. Ketoconazole 200mg po qd-bid for 6 months d. Fluconazole 150mg po qwk for up to 12 months e. Griseofulvin 250-375 mg ultramicrosized (500mg po microsized) po bid for 4-9 months for fingernails, 6-18 months for toenails
	2. Surgical or chemical nail plate avulsion followed by topical antifungal therapy

F. Tinea Versicolor	1. Mild/localized cases
	a. Ketoconazole or selenium sulfide or zinc pyrithione or sulfur shampoos
	2. Widespread/recalcitrant disease
	a. Ketoconazole 200mg po qd for one week or 400mg po x1, repeat in one week b. Itraconazole 200mg po qd for one week c. Fluconazole 400mg po x1

G. Candidiasis (Intertrigo)	1. Mild/localized cases
	a. Nystatin or imidazole preparations (econazole, ketoconazole, etc.) b. Gentian violet or thymol preparations **keep area dry with powder (Zeabsorb) and aerated
	2. Severe/recalcitrant cases
	a. Ketoconazole 200mg po qd for 1-2 weeks b. Itraconazole 100mg po qd for 3-12 weeks c. Fluconazole 50mg po qd

Dedoncker, P et al. Pulse therapy with one-week itraconazole monthly for three or four months in the treatment of onychomycosis. Cutis 1995;56:180-3.
Gupta, AK et al. Antifungal agents: An Overview. Part 1. J Am Acad Dermatol. 1994;30:677-98.
Gupta, AK et al. Antifungal agents: An Overview. Part 2. J Am Acad Dermatol. 1994;30:911-33.